Letters to a New Vegan

Carol J. Adams

Living among Meat Eaters

The Vegetarian's Survival Handbook

336 pp, 978-1-59056-116-4, paperback

A. Breeze Harper, Editor

Sistah Vegan

Black Female Vegans Speaks on Food, Identity, Health, and Society

224 pp, 978-1-59056-145-4, paperback

Victorian Moran

The Love-Powered Diet

Eating for Freedom, Health, and Joy

264 pp, 978-1-59056-117-1, paperback

Pamela Rice

101 Reasons Why I'm a Vegetarian

288 pp, 978-1-59056-075-4, paperback

Will Tuttle

The World Peace Diet

Eating for Spiritual Health and Social Harmony

352 pp, 978-1-59056-083-9, paperback

LETTERS *to a* NEW VEGAN

Words to Inform, Inspire,
and Support a Vegan Lifestyle

Lantern Books • New York
A Division of Booklight Inc.

2015

Lantern Books

128 Second Place

Brooklyn, NY 11231

www.lanternbooks.com

Printed in the United States of America

Library of Congress Cataloging-in-Publication Data

Letters to a new vegan : words to inform, inspire,
and support a vegan lifestyle.
      pages cm
   ISBN 978-1-59056-504-9 (paperback : alk. paper)—
ISBN 978-1-59056-505-6 (ebook)
   1. Veganism—Miscellanea. I. Lantern Books.
   TX392.L493 2015
   613.2'622--dc23

                              2014049786

Introduction

Martin Rowe

Editor-in-Chief at Lantern Books

In 2014, a scholar of literature and long-time vegan contacted me with a proposal. She told me how, when she was in college, a friend had given her *Letters to a Young Poet* by the Czech writer Rainer Maria Rilke. From Rilke's slim volume, published three years after his death in 1926, a particular passage had stayed with her over the years:

> Be patient toward all that is unsolved in your heart and try to love the questions themselves, like locked rooms and like books that are now written in a very foreign tongue. Do not now seek the answers, which cannot be given you because you would not be able to live them. And the point is, to live

everything. Live the questions now. Perhaps you will then gradually, without noticing it, live along some distant day into the answer.

"That's exactly how I found my own way to veganism," she said. "By living the questions."

Just as Rilke felt compelled to advise a nineteen-year-old following in his footsteps on the intellectual, psychological, and practical requirements of a life dedicated to poetry, so Melissa Tedrowe had the idea of inviting those who'd committed themselves to veganism to mentor others starting out on that path. As with Rilke, the advice would take the form of a letter, in this case to an anonymous friend, with the aim of not only offering wisdom, encouragement, and counsel, but showing the newly minted vegan the varieties of experiences and influences of others who no longer ate or wore animal products, and who were advocates for the welfare and rights of nonhuman beings.

The idea struck us at Lantern as compelling. Our publishing company has produced many books over the years on veganism and animal advocacy, the majority of which focus on strategy and the philosophy behind social change—in other words, reasons why one should become a vegan and how to persuade others to take that step. Where we (and perhaps many others within the animal advocacy or vegan movements) may not have been diligent enough is in providing suggestions on how to *remain* a vegan.

Just how poorly we were doing was confirmed by a 2014 survey of 11,000 adults in the United States. The survey, conducted by the Humane Research Council, found that two percent of respondents identified themselves as vegan or vegetarian; 88 percent had never given up animal products; and 10 percent considered themselves *former* vegetarians or vegans. This news caused many of us among the two percent to do some soul-searching. How was it that after so many years, so few of us were vegan or vegetarian? And, even more gallingly, how could 84 percent of vegans and vegetarians return to an omnivorous diet?

The survey offered some answers: 63 percent of former vegans and vegetarians started eating meat because they didn't like standing out from the crowd; almost half of them felt they had had "insufficient interaction" with other vegans or vegetarians; and 58 percent decided that their diet was not "part of their identity." Intriguingly, however, of those who had gone back to consuming animal products, almost

40 percent were interested in returning to veganism or vegetarianism. This last statistic, suggested the survey's authors, revealed that for many people, veganism or vegetarianism was proving logistically, dietetically, or socially complicated. If a means could be found, they added, to make it easier or more socially acceptable, the number of vegans or vegetarians in the U. S. could triple.

The concept of *Letters to a New Vegan*, therefore, couldn't have been timelier. Many of us who decide to reduce our personal role in the exploitation of animals experience a profound shift in how we relate to the world. Sometimes, this movement is traumatic; sometimes, it isn't. Much of the time, it's a mixture of exhilaration and despair, confusion and relief. What often makes a difference is the support and solidarity of others—a friend or colleague who can help you not to feel quite so alone. Justin Van Kleeck, who later joined Melissa in the editing process, suggested that, like the traditional *vade mecum* books, *Letters to a New Vegan* could be a companion volume that would "go with you" always, anywhere, and perhaps, in its small way, help to reduce the percentage of those who return to omnivorism as well as bring more people to the cause.

So, working with Melissa and Justin, we

gathered the collection you hold here. We were thrilled at the overwhelming response to our call for contributions. Although we realized that the vegan community was growing around the globe (recidivism notwithstanding), we could not and did not expect such widespread interest in connecting through the ancient familiarity of the letter. It was humbling, to say the least, and gave us great pride in our shared community.

The sheer number of offerings also made the selection process difficult. Ultimately, however, we relied on a variety of typical editorial criteria including clarity, strength of voice, tightness, and originality. However, we also strove for a diversity of voices, based on geography, gender, age, and other demographic factors. We didn't set parameters around what it means to be a "new" vegan, leaving that choice up to our contributors.

One criterion, however, did unify the selections we chose: implicitly or explicitly, they each affirmed the original definition of veganism developed by Donald Watson and The Vegan Society in 1944:

> The word "veganism" denotes a philosophy and way of living which seeks to exclude—as far as is possible

and practical—all forms of exploitation of, and cruelty to, animals for food, clothing or any other purpose; and by extension, promotes the development and use of animal-free alternatives for the benefit of humans, animals and the environment. In dietary terms it denotes the practice of dispensing with all products derived wholly or partly from animals.

Watson's definition balances negative (exclusion) with positive (promotion and development), while affirming the central tenet of ending human violence toward, and exploitation of, our fellow living beings. It speaks volumes about the vital importance of an ethical approach to nonhuman life that, as the 2014 survey discovered, more than two-thirds of those who remain vegan or vegetarian do so as part of a commitment to animal protection.

Like all anthologies, the selection in *Letters to a New Vegan* is necessarily partial and imperfect. Nonetheless, we hope you'll agree that together these words constitute a powerfully sustaining message from vegans, to vegans—one that can help a vibrantly compassionate veganism not just endure but thrive. We at Lantern are thankful for Melissa and Justin's original vision, and, of course, for all those who contributed to this volume.

—*Martin Rowe*
Brooklyn, New York
May 2015

Dear New Vegan,

It may seem that nobody else shares your enthusiasm about the change you have just made in your life. You have decided to sacrifice your taste buds in order to create the largest single reduction in the consumption of natural resources that you personally can make, the healthiest choice you can make for your body, and the biggest way to reduce violence and slavery while promoting peace in the world, all with one simple lifestyle change. (Plus, those taste buds are going to change in just a few weeks, and you aren't going to be missing cheese anymore. Trust me!) Nobody else around you might realize it yet, but you are an incredible example of what our world can become in the future.

Remember, though, not to become a junk-food vegan who lives on potato chips and Oreos. If you stick to it, you are going to fall in love (perhaps again) with vegetables, fruit, beans, and other whole plant foods because they are going to make your body feel great and you will finally realize how delicious they actually taste naturally. And remember to always take a B_{12} supplement! If you find that you are hungry all the time, then just eat more until you are full, as plants generally are less calorie dense and you need to eat more of them than you would have on your old diet.

Be proud of the choice you have made and continue to make each day, share your reasons for it with others, but also realize that many others aren't as far along on the path as you are. Encourage them even if they can only make small changes in the right direction at the moment. If you are willing to accept where others are, encourage them to follow the same path, and constantly radiate joy from the vegan lifestyle that you continually choose, then you will be surprised at whom you actually influence and who also decides to follow you down that path. Then, your already monumentally positive change will be multiplied and will ripple out into those around you. You are truly changing the world for the better.

Congratulations on making one of the simplest yet most powerful changes in your life and the world we live in. You are an amazing human being!

Keane Southard
Northborough, Massachusetts

Dear New Vegan,

If you're like me, you've always loved animals. From Old MacDonald to *Charlotte's Web*, didn't we both grow up hearing nursery songs and reading books about the wonders of the animal world?

I'm not really sure when I seemed to lose my way. How did I change? How did I lose that early connection to animals? I drank milk, not knowing a baby calf died for that glass of milk. I ate eggs, not knowing billions of male chicks were killed because they were of no use. I savored my cheese, not knowing a cow was artificially inseminated by force (what some might call rape) so she could be kept constantly pregnant. I enjoyed lox on a bagel, oblivious to all the marine life dying in mile-long nets in order for the more popular fish to be caught.

I had so easily swallowed the "Happy Cow" and "Got Milk?" and "Meat = Protein" advertising campaigns, never questioning the truth for the animals behind the slogans. One day, stuck in a traffic jam next to a truck loaded with thousands of caged chickens, I felt them all looking at me. They appealed to the child within: "Why have you forsaken us?"

From that day forward, I vowed to become a vegan.

I welcome you as a new vegan to this world you knew as a child—i.e., the world of revering animals. I won't lie. Now that you're an adult, it won't be easy. You'll face ridicule from those still wearing blinders. For some, it seems to be the way they cope with their chosen lifestyle. Above all, it will be a challenge to remain calm and polite. You will be made an example of, and it will be up to you to be a role model and spokesperson for the animals. They are the voiceless. You are their voice.

You'll need to educate yourself with facts. Whether you like it or not, people will expect you to defend your position. Ironically, they don't see the need to defend the torture their lifestyle promotes. As you look deeper into the real world of factory farming and agriculture, it will shock and depress you. It will be hard to stay positive, but you must.

Focus on the good stories: the sanctuaries doing wonderful rescue work, the shelter adoptions, the growing number of animal advocates speaking up, the vegan celebrities stepping up. Sometimes, focusing on the individual stories is more beneficial than focusing on the bigger picture. It truly helps to keep you positive in a world you'll often think has gone mad.

Don't kid yourself: the journey is long. As a new vegan, you'll be amazed at how much you didn't know. We're drowning in animal products, and we've been oblivious. Take it slowly, but keep moving forward, eliminating more and more animal products from your life. It's not all or nothing; it's a progression.

Don't let anyone criticize you for taking your time along this journey. The important thing is the huge difference you, and you alone, are making by reconnecting with the animals you always knew you loved.

When a friend notices how much better you seem as a vegan—that's a win. When you share a vegan dish and someone says, "Hey, this tastes good!"— that's a win. When your health tests come back better than ever—that's a win. When you celebrate a cruelty-free, traditional holiday with your family— that's a win. When you weed out the leather or fur jackets, belts, and bags from your closet—that's a win. When you walk through a grocery store and spend most of your time in the produce section— that's a win. Celebrate each and every one of these milestones!

One day, this will all seem "normal" to you. The best day is when you see a pig and you don't see bacon. Instead, you can't help but flash back to that childhood memory of Charlotte saving Wilbur, the pig. Or you hear a cow mooing and you don't think of steak. Instead, you smile as the tune of Old MacDonald plays softly in your head.

That's when you know your life has come full circle and you've finally become who you knew you were all along—a compassionate human being.

For the animals always,

Julie Hanan
Highlands Ranch, Colorado

3

Dear New Vegan,

Congratulations on doing the single most important thing most of us can do to improve our health, protect the environment, and reduce the number of other animals hurt and killed every year by us humans.

I have been vegan since the summer of 1972. When I became a vegan, *vegan* wasn't a word I knew. Today, I see the word everywhere.

For me, the hardest part of adopting a vegan lifestyle was the indifference I discovered in the people I cared the most for at the time. It was difficult as a new vegan to see that no one else seemed to understand why I had decided to stop eating animals—eating eggs, milk, cheese, honey, and the rest—and wearing fur and leather. No matter how many times we talked about it, it was like I was speaking a different language. My friends were polite and accommodating when we ate together, but beyond that they were dead to the concerns that motivated me to change my behavior so radically.

After many years, nearly twenty years in some cases, I simply gave up on them. I still have hope for them, but the disappointment of having very close long-term friends not seeming to care very much about the harm they were (are) causing was finally just too much.

Over time, I made new friends. I discovered a large planet-wide community of like-minded people. I still speak to non-vegans regularly about the benefits of a vegan lifestyle, but now I'm talking to people I generally don't know while tabling or handing out leaflets. I have great hope for them as well, but I'm not emotionally invested in what they think.

So, good luck. You aren't alone. There are lots of people who get it and are thrilled that you get it, too.

Rick Bogle
Madison, Wisconsin

4

Dear New Vegan,

You are wonderful!

I remember my first morning as a vegan after being vegetarian for many years. I finally felt those last bits of sadness and guilt leave my shoulders. I felt lighter and happier and more at peace.

That was sixteen years ago, before the word *vegan* was as well known as it is today, so there weren't a lot of vegan products available. I feel fortunate that I became vegan then, because today when I look at all of the vegan merchandise, I get a little overwhelmed.

Maybe you feel that way now—overwhelmed. Here are four random suggestions that may help you during your first days, weeks, or months of being vegan:

- First of all, feel good about what you are doing. You will be happier and healthier, and will no longer be contributing to the suffering of animals raised for food. That is huge!
- Find one or two good vegan cookbooks and work through them

before buying more. For years, the only vegan cookbook I had was *Vegan Vittles* by Joan Stepaniak, and I go back to that one quite often. Now I've expanded to *The Joy of Vegan Baking* and *The Vegan Table* by Colleen Patrick-Goudreau. Those three cookbooks and an abundance of online recipes are all I use. Remember that cookbooks come from trees. Keep your consumption low. It all adds up for the animals and for the planet.

- Get to know the easy replacements for eggs. With that one bit of information you can still enjoy your mother's favorite chocolate cake recipe or your favorite pancake recipe. There are lists online, and there is also a wonderful egg replacement poster available on Etsy. I have one on my refrigerator.

- Family members are the hardest to convince. Accept the fact that they may not change, ever. Love them anyway.

Keep in mind that being vegan is not difficult. It's really simple. You can do it.

Lynn Pauly
Madison, Wisconsin

5

Dear New Vegan,

Food has significant cultural value. For thousands of years humans have gathered together to share meals and celebrate special days and rituals with food. The importance of food to culture is so strong in some traditions that it is seen as an offense to refuse it. While the transition for new vegans is difficult enough—learning to read labels, learning how to cook differently, adjusting shopping and eating habits, finding new restaurants—the additional cultural aspect of eating can have severe implications.

It was many years ago, in 1998, when I first decided that I could no longer support an industry that harms animals. I was sixteen, and while my own family adjusted empathetically to my decision, there were many awkward meals with strangers, many awkward dinners with new friends, and many terrible potato-chip-and-mustard sandwiches. Even today there are occasional feelings of ridicule in the glances and questions of those around me at dinner tables.

The question is bound to come up. Your partner invites you over for dinner with her family. She tells her parents you are a vegan. They ask why. She gives them an answer. Her parents, being good hosts, make a special side dish that vegans can eat—mashed potatoes. You attend the dinner. Everything is going fine. The food is served, but you see a canister of butter on the counter. You ask, "Is there butter in the mashed potatoes?" Her parents answer, "Yes," as the entire table suddenly realizes that you can't (won't) eat most of what was prepared. You apologize, but maybe you brought a vegan side dish and your own act of cultural food sharing is enough to diffuse the situation. The question is still bound to come up: "Why? Why are you a vegan?"

Answering a question like this in such a moment is like navigating a rowboat through a minefield. I've given many answers in the last fifteen years: "It's better for the environment," "There are lots of reasons but it makes me feel healthier," "There is no reason not to," "I can't bring myself to contribute to factory farming," or my personal favorite, "I started to see all animals in the way most people see dogs— as beings. When I see a cow or a pig I simply don't see food—I see beings." None of these answers feel satisfactory. All of them bring you out of the dietary closet as different, as other. And while no one has said it to my face, I feel it in their glances, their tones, their defensiveness, their dismissal. It's even hinted at in their acceptance: you are different.

Of all the struggles and difficulties in my first years of the vegan lifestyle, alienation was the most difficult. Even when people were kind and welcoming, they were kind and welcoming to someone who did not participate in the same cultural food rituals as they did. I still felt isolated at most gatherings. While I now live in a major metropolitan area with a community of kindred spirits and a plethora of vegan-friendly restaurants, it wasn't always like this. I didn't know a single other vegetarian in the small town where I grew up, and "vegan-friendly" restaurants usually meant pizza without the cheese or plain bean burritos. As it was, I didn't actually meet another vegetarian until six years after my transition. I didn't meet another vegan until eight years after my transition.

How do you overcome feelings of alienation as a new vegan?

The obvious solution is to surround yourself with a kindred community. Did you know that the percentage of vegans in the United States has gone up from one to two percent in the last five years? Although meeting other vegans can be difficult in some regions, with the advent of the Internet and the growing popularity of vegetarianism and veganism in general, the number of sites acting as meeting spaces or facilitating vegan gatherings has grown exponentially. Simply reading common experiences on a forum can ease feelings of alienation, and was one of the first ways I reached out to the vegan community writ large. But the other, not as obvious, answer to the burden of alienation and othering is to be mindful of the large historical contingent of those who have cared for animals. Sometimes a simple reminder that great people eschewed the eating of animal flesh is all it takes to ease the binds of alienation from the heart.

My advice to you, new vegan, is to seek out these historical and contemporary connections in addition to the community groups and meet-ups around your place of residence. Veganism as a paradigm of showing compassion toward animals existed several millennia before Donald Watson coined the term "vegan" in 1944. This is not a recent fad. Know that you are in good company, even when eating a chip sandwich at a table of cheeseburgers. Your kindred are many in number. Although evidence varies, the following are believed to be vegetarian and/or vegan by many historians: Gautama Buddha, Leonardo Da Vinci, Plutarch, Porphyry, Pythagoras,

George Bernard Shaw, St. Basil the Great, St. Isaac the Syrian, St. John Chrysostom, Percy Shelley, Leo Tolstoy, John Wesley, Ellen G. White, and William Wilberforce. Look around and you'll see many contemporary counterparts. You also have all the wonderful writers in this book, all the animals you stopped eating, and many others to call friend. When the feelings of alienation begin to burden your life, know that your kindred are many and that your name has a place next to theirs.

Jason Derry
Denver, Colorado

6

Dear New Vegan,

Welcome! Perhaps you have been vegetarian for a while or experimented with veganism earlier in your life. Perhaps you knew it was better for you, but you felt that it isolated you from social eating with friends and family. Today you will find many more vegan restaurant choices and reasonably priced vegan choices in most markets. You will be amazed at how many vegan cookbooks, prepared products, and ingredients are easily available to you. Almost any of your favorite meat dishes and comfort foods can be easily veganized.

You may be worried that you will feel hungry and deprived, and have nothing to eat. You need not fear. You are entering a world of rich flavor, healthy nourishment for your body, and the satisfaction of helping to heal our Earth and promote the just treatment of other living beings.

I became a vegetarian at age fifty. I knew intellectually that the meat on my plate was animal flesh, but when I finally admitted to myself the suffering these animals endured, meat was no longer possible for me. I had health concerns that also motivated my change to a meat-free diet, but when these resolved I realized I felt so much better eating this way and felt it was more aligned with my ethics, so I continued. I explored new meals to cook. I lost twenty pounds.

Several years later, again for health and ethical reasons, I decided to become vegan. It was easier than I expected. I made low-fat choices and lost another thirty-five pounds. I staved off impending diabetes.

You can choose to get into discussions with friends and family, or not. You do not have to explain your choice to be vegan, but doing so can be an opportunity to educate. I have found discussions at mealtimes to be useless; they tend to be argumentative, defensive, and only a means for others to rationalize what is on their plates. Any real dialogue is best saved for another setting.

Make friends with other vegans. Share meals and ideas; enjoy validation for dessert.

Enjoy how good your body feels.

Know you are caring for our Earth.

Realize you are showing others healthier possibilities by your example.

Appreciate that fewer animals are suffering because of you and that you are not taking their suffering into your body and mind.

Any change takes time to get used to. So be patient, and gather what you need to succeed. You will be amazed at how possible this is and how good you feel. Step into your power! Rejoice!

This is my advice to you as a new vegan.

Shelley Kaplan
Salem, Oregon

Dear New Vegan,

I wholeheartedly thank my omnivorous parents for being honest with me about the origins of my meals and allowing me to make my own food choices at such a young age. I have been a vegetarian since age two out of a deep-seated aversion to consuming animals. Since then I've continued to learn about the meat and dairy industries and have replaced all animal products from my diet (and wardrobe) with ethical, plant-based alternatives.

Take my word for it: There is something personal to gain from acknowledging the discrepancy between your everyday food choices and your personal values. It just takes a bit of education on the one hand and soul searching on the other. Identifying what in this world is important to me has been grounding. And living true to my heart is sincerely uplifting.

I am, by no stretch, a foodie. Everything I cook is easy, which is the third requirement for my food next to vegan (first) and yummy (second). I'm also not a health fanatic, though I'm health aware and seek to avoid deficiencies. I'm glad flax seeds are full of omega-3s, and I use them because it is the easiest and yummiest way to replace eggs in my baking. What I care about most is the ethical treatment of human and nonhuman animals.

Shadrup and I have decided to raise our children vegan. This means that we teach them to make mindful everyday decisions, emphasizing the wellbeing of others alongside meeting our own needs. My four-year-old son Amdo and nine-year-old daughter Ruby are influenced, but decidedly not forced, by our choice to be vegan. If it is not a heartfelt decision on their part to refrain from eating certain foods (many of which appear to be treats to a child), my fear is they will develop resentment toward the vegan diet and food will become an issue of control rather than a point of connection and dialogue.

Ruby cannot bring non-vegan food to her lips in light of the immense suffering of the animals. I say that with unparalleled pride. How did this come to pass? I've taken Ruby to visit an animal sanctuary in Woodstock, New York, for years, and now that she is old enough, we go to volunteer. She has read a lot of vegan literature. She has met Jenny Brown—activist, author, and co-founder of Woodstock Farm Animal Sanctuary—on several occasions. Jenny encourages her to follow her compassionate heart.

Amdo talks a lot about the suffering of animals, but when he is eating with people outside of our immediate family he often chooses to eat non-vegan foods. When I am present, I offer him vegan alternatives but never let his emotions elevate to a level of distress. I am confident he will grow into a critical thinker and come to sensible and sustainable lifestyle choices, especially with the backdrop of unconditional love from his family. We don't want to face the boomerang effect. Amdo is comfortable saying, "My family is vegan, but it's my choice and sometimes I pick non-vegan foods."

I love the example that I am setting for my kids and their friends. I am outwardly cool but inwardly gushing as I watch my little loves observe this world through an ethical lens. My relationships with friends, family, and children are strong and clear because I know who I am and feel good about the choices I make. I've been told by some close friends that my being vegan makes them feel guilty or in fear of my judgment. It shouldn't matter whether I judge. My answer to them is: The only person who has to feel good about the way you eat is you. If my dietary choices make you uncomfortable, then maybe you don't feel a hundred percent confident in your choices and need to investigate and think them through some more. I won't say anything unsolicited, but I certainly won't pretend not to care what people eat just to make them feel more comfortable. Sorry!

Lara Goodman
New York, New York

7B

Dear New Vegan,

My name is Ruby and I am nine years old. I interviewed some of my classmates about how much they love animals. They answered on a scale of 1 to 10. Most kids loved animals at 9 and 10. One girl even said she loved animals at a 15! I asked them many questions about foods they like to eat. When I got home I put all my information on a chart inside my notebook. I looked for which animal lovers were vegan, and there were none. They all (and I mean *all*) answered "yes" to the question, "Do you like cheese and crackers?" I checked for vegetarian animal lovers, and there was only one. I think if she understood what was going on she would be a vegan, too. I remember that one of my classmates said she loves animals but can't stop eating meat because she wouldn't know what else to eat. One girl said she didn't want to eat meat but wasn't allowed to stop. Some grown-ups I know say they want to stop, but they think they can't, like being addicted to cigarettes. I want to learn about the block between wanting to stop but just not doing it.

I am a very proud vegan because I am not supporting something that I don't believe in. I am glad that you are trying to do that, too.

Ruby Goodman
New York, New York

8

Dear New Vegan,

Three years ago, I was on one of my cross-country motorcycle trips. Making our way back to Chicago, my buddy and I stopped at the Thurman Café in Columbus, Ohio. I had a mission: I had seen on TV, and now wanted to attempt to eat, the Thurmanator, a foot-high and nearly three-pound burger. An hour and a half later, mission accomplished! On another occasion, I ate nine brats at a baseball game (one per inning). On a dare, I once ate thirty-six wings in twenty minutes. Three years ago, I ate twenty-two tamales at a Cinco de Mayo party. Gluttony!

On January 17, 2012, almost on a whim, I decided to try a vegetarian diet, still without a whit of concern for the plight of the animals. I just thought it would be cool and probably healthy. A day or two into my new diet, a Facebook friend suggested I watch *Earthlings*. I didn't know what it was about, but I had an idea. I put it off at first, but five days into my vegetarian experiment, I decided it was time to watch it. I hopped up on my elliptical, turned on my computer, and started watching.

Twenty minutes later, I was muttering, "No, no, no." Ten minutes later, to no one in particular, I was saying, "Stop, please, stop." Five minutes later, sweat and tears streaming down my face, I was a vegan. It was January 22, 2012. I didn't even know how to pronounce the word, but I knew my life had changed.

The change was profound. I immediately felt much happier and lighter as I walked around this world knowing that I was doing my part in preventing animal suffering. I had seen what humans do to animals. I would not hurt an animal, and I will not pay to have people do it for me. It is wrong. It is cruel.

I have a choice. I won't take part in it anymore. And I haven't given up a thing. In fact, I have more choices in food, more freedom from advertisers, and an amazing liberation from lazy thinking.

We have had many pets. In my case, we have loved Maynard, Twiggy, Simon, Gretel, Angel, Priscilla, Easter, Barouk, Abby, Dayna, Sugar, Penny, Jenny, Gellie, Sneakers, Raisen, Debris, Cookie, Pharaoh, Augee, Dustee, Tom, Roxie, Oliver, Louie, and Henry. Each one had or has their individual personality. Similarly, each pig, cow, chicken, elephant, sheep, deer, turkey, duck, goose, and fish also has a personality. They are individuals. And they feel pain. They can and do suffer.

You can be a "dog lover" or a "cat person" or a birdwatcher. However, you cannot truly be an "animal lover" if you eat meat. Interestingly enough, you don't have to love animals to be vegan. I don't love all animals, just as I don't love all human beings. I respect all animals and their rights as individuals. They have exactly the same right to live their lives, from their point of view, as we do. Animals are innocent.

The things we do in order to stock our refrigerators, cabinets, and closets are brutal. Animals are in misery. They suffer through a shortened and horrible life.

And then they are executed—unloved, scared, and without any dignity. The suffering that each animal has to endure should make us wince.

We can change all of that. Being vegan is as easy or as hard as you make it. It takes an open mind and the willingness to rethink what you have always believed. We don't need meat, cheese, eggs, and dairy. We like these things, but no, we definitely do not need them. We buy them because we always have. We buy because that's what we have been told to do by the government, by advertisers, and by our parents. We buy because: 1) we think it's easy; 2) we think it tastes good; and 3) we think it's cheaper.

But it's none of those.

Over the past two and a half years, I have read at least twenty books on topics ranging from nutrition and health to animal rights and ethics. I don't know everything, but I do know that the way we treat animals is wrong. I know it is easy to ignore ugly truths. It is hard to face ideas that go against what we believe. I also know that none of us is too old to try new things, or to change.

It is important for you to do your own research. It helps to be confident and prepared for the inevitable, often tiresome questions from those around you. It is important to respond calmly, with facts and the strong, quiet grace that comes from knowing that what you are doing is helping make this world a better place for all.

Mark Turner
Chicago, Illinois

9

Dear New Vegan,

Though I have never met you, in many ways I believe we already know each other very well. Our struggles have not been identical, yet I am sure we have shared many. The world is a tough place to live in, especially for a person who chooses not to follow the path of least resistance. This is why I am writing you this letter: to tell you to never give up.

Fear is a weapon used to keep change from happening, effectively halting progress. Fear comes at you from all directions: from the government, giant corporations, your teachers, your friends, your family, and even yourself. They will tell you: "You are just one person. What difference could you possibly make?" "What you're doing is far too difficult." And, "Your actions will get you into trouble." Sometimes, no matter how long you've been in the game, you can feel as though you will succumb to those negative thoughts simply because they never stop.

They replay constantly in your mind, dragging you down until you stand petrified—paralyzed by fear. This is exactly what they want.

You may feel alone. You may feel hopeless. You

may feel as though the entire world is against you. You may feel as though giving up would be so much simpler and easier than continuing to fight. These are feelings every activist has wrestled with.

I won't lie to you and tell you that these feelings will ever completely disappear. The truth is, they are always there in the shadows of your mind, waiting for the moment you are most vulnerable to present themselves. They grow and fester like a disease in your psyche, whose symptoms go unnoticed at first but in time grow to become unbearable and impossible to ignore.

This is the life you have chosen. The feeling of loneliness in a crowded room—of existing separate from the rest—is something that will remain constant. Seeing life as it really is, rather than the façade you were brought up to not question or look past, will haunt you at every turn. It is a life of conflict, of grief, and often of solitude.

But it is also a life of gratitude, joy, and boundless love. It is a life of honesty and integrity. It is a life characterized by your unwillingness to turn a blind eye to suffering. It is a life of purpose beyond the self.

This world needs people like you—people who are willing to speak the truth no matter where they are or who is listening. People who are willing to act. People who always eagerly ask, "How can I do more?" Because the truth is, these are the only people who have ever changed the tides of history. The world is full of bystanders, those who see injustice happening right in front of them and are too afraid to stop it, who think, "Someone ought to do something about this," and do not do something about it themselves. The world needs people like you, who will take a stand against injustice and oppression.

I would not ask you to be fearless. To be fearless is to be reckless and in this context is not only unwise but also nearly impossible. Instead, what I am asking of you is to be courageous.

Courage is not the lack of fear, but the willingness to overcome it.

Fear seeks to control—to immobilize. In this life you have to learn to challenge your fears so that you can overcome them. You have to be willing to venture out of your comfort zone, do what needs to be done, and be willing to accept the consequences. The satisfaction you will get from knowing you are true to your beliefs in times of conflict and uncertainty will far outweigh any negativity you might encounter.

So, dear friend, though you do not know me,

have never met me, and likely never will, take some comfort in knowing that even from separate ends of the Earth, I am here fighting right beside you, pushing you to be better and, most importantly, steadfastly believing in our cause: the cause of total animal liberation. We must believe, and we must persevere, because to give up means that fear has won. And that is something people like you and me do not allow.

"Few are willing to brave the disapproval of their fellows, the censure of their colleagues, the wrath of their society. Moral courage is a rarer commodity than bravery in battle or great intelligence. Yet it is the one essential, vital quality for those who seek to change a world that yields most painfully to change."—Robert F. Kennedy

Kara Kapelnikova
Los Angeles, California

10

Dear New Vegan,

I wonder what brought you here? Did you watch *Forks Over Knives* or one of the other works extolling the growing evidence of the many health benefits of veganism? Did you watch too many videos about the cruelty of factory farming on YouTube? Maybe you have a beloved pet and you became uncomfortable with our culture's norm of raising some animals to kill and eat while raising others as loved family members. I've been through all of these experiences and stages of thought, and they brought me to the same point as you just a few years ago.

It's an exciting time to be a vegan! There are more vegan food options than ever before, and the acceptance of this lifestyle is accelerating quickly. You can comfortably eat almost anywhere you go. You'll find that restricting your diet paradoxically leads you to a world of new flavors and discoveries.

My advice for you: Get a few vegan cookbooks. We like the *Forks Over Knives* cookbook as well as the many Internet resources for vegan recipes. Embrace the new spices and dishes. They might be foreign to you, but you'll be so glad that you learned about them. Soon, returning to the "Standard American Diet" won't even cross your mind

Be excited and committed to your new lifestyle but don't give way to judgment and preachiness towards others. Providing someone with information and creating some interesting, challenging dialogue is often welcomed, but it's easy and self-serving to look down on others. Continue to educate yourself. It will constantly reinforce your willpower to learn more about the new discoveries about the benefits of veganism. I enjoy watching nutritionfacts.org for this.

Join the vegan community. Go to some local vegan cooking classes, keep up with some vegan Facebook communities, and cook your friends some awesome food and convert them the right way!

Good luck and enjoy the journey,

Kurt Schwemmer
Colorado Springs, Colorado

11

Dear New Vegan,

I remember the moment I seriously wondered about the animal on my plate. I was a small child. I noticed the discomfort in the adults around me when I asked about it. Their eyes darted at each other; they were suddenly at a loss for words. My father's voice filled the silence: "It's your dinner. Eat it." His tone implied there would be consequences, painful ones, if I didn't . . . so I did. When I got my grandmother alone, I asked her to please tell me. She said: "Well . . . cows give us milk and hamburgers and roast beef. Pigs give us pork chops and bacon. Chickens give us eggs and chicken breasts and drumsticks. Turkeys give us, well, turkey."

I thought about that. In my heart, I felt the warm benevolence of these animals. Still, I was troubled. I couldn't figure out exactly how the cow gave us a hamburger. Did she have a special "hamburger hole" in her body? Did a roast grow on their backs like huge lumps until they fell off in the fields with the farmers wandering around collecting them? I went back to my grandma and told her my theories. After relentless persistence on my part, she finally told me.

I was horrified. My picture books showed mother hens protecting and teaching their chicks. In my coloring books, I carefully stayed within the lines with my pink crayon as the pig smiled at my efforts from the page. A milk carton had a picture of a happy cow. All lies. All illusion. And *everybody* was in on it! Even the kind people who loved me. Even myself. I told my parents I wouldn't eat anything that came from an animal. I said: "They didn't give it to us. We hurt them and kill them and steal it from them. You told me not to be a stealer." I was told I would do what I was told . . . and I did.

Innocence is lost in pieces. Fear of my father's violence overrode my own inner voice. Acting in opposition to what I felt and knew was right made me a killer by proxy, a coward, a small speck in a raging sea, without an oar, drifting. . . .

What is lost can be found, however.

Flash forward. I am a college student. I am a registered nurse. Over the years, my family has included dogs, cats, rabbits, birds, guinea pigs, and a hedgehog, in addition to four biological children. I am a busy mother, mostly drifting through life, when my child asks me about the animal on her plate. Something inside of me stirs, comes unmoored, as I am faced with my own childhood question being asked by my child. Without hesitation, I tell her the truth. She says she wants no part of that. I say: "OK." She asks me why my actions don't match my beliefs. I tell her: "I don't know." She says I taught her to know those things about herself.

In a simple, beautiful, deeply profound way, her question awakened me. My actions moved purposefully into alignment with the voice of my heart and soul and truth. Going vegan was my becoming. I am who I want to be in this world.

New Vegan, I'm grateful to the path inside you that led you here.

With Peace,

Tracy Curtis
Anoka, Minnesota

12

Dear New Vegan,

I welcome you warmly to the growing community of people who are choosing to eat and live compassionately. As you begin your vegan life, you may feel at first that your choice is a difficult one, perhaps too difficult at times. But I urge you to stay true to your decision, because it is the right one. I became vegan in 1983 after being vegetarian for ten years, never realizing, during those years, that dairy milk and eggs are every bit as much a part of an animal's body as meat is, and that hens and cows and their young are treated just as badly as, and are eventually slaughtered the same as, animals raised for meat.

I will tell you, briefly, why I stopped eating meat, and, finally, all animal products. I grew up in a meat-eating household in Pennsylvania. Although I always loved animals, I ate animal products so unthinkingly that I would argue with my father against hunting at the dinner table over a plateful of once-living creatures who at that time were invisible to me as having recently been animals.

In the 1970s I discovered an essay by the Russian writer Leo Tolstoy in which he vividly described his visits to Moscow slaughterhouses. Having witnessed those scenes of suffering, he urged that the first step toward a compassionate, nonviolent life is to get the animal bloodshed out of one's system. I immediately quit eating meat. Later, philosopher Peter Singer's book *Animal Liberation* and a cookbook called *The Cookbook for People Who Love Animals* opened my eyes to the truth of dairy and eggs, and I saw I could no longer ethically consume those products.

For many new vegans, including me, cheese was the biggest hurdle, but I got over it. One day, I sat in my car in front of my favorite Italian restaurant in College Park, Maryland, crying because I could no longer have pizza with extra (or any!) cheese. I had a good cry in the driver's seat. Then I dried my eyes, went inside, ordered rigatoni with mushrooms, and never looked back.

I wish that in childhood I had made the connection between eating and animals, but I didn't. As a child growing up in a community where schools were (and still are) closed on the first day of hunting season, where ring-necked pheasants are pen-raised to be released into the woods to be shot for pleasure by hunters, I hated those things, yet I didn't think about animals in relation to the dinner table. While

I don't hold myself responsible for what I didn't realize at the time, once my eyes were open, I was responsible.

To this day I consider my decision to keep faith with animals by respecting them and not eating them to be the single best decision I have ever made. For me, being vegan is the opposite of renunciation and "doing without." It is a totally positive, deeply satisfying diet and dietary decision that has influenced my attitude and behavior in other areas, including household and personal care products, and in trying to act consciously instead of just conveniently.

If I have any advice to give, it is to stay firm in your commitment and be happy about it. Practically speaking, I would encourage you to eat a wholesome vegan diet and not gorge solely on vegan junk food. I would encourage you to educate yourself about vegan nutrition and to share what you are learning with others in a friendly way. Offer to cook a family dinner once a week (or more), make sure that what you serve is delicious, and do everything possible to make being vegan an affirmative, pleasurable, and fulfilling experience. Remember the animals whose lives you are no longer ruining just for a meal. For me, this is the most powerful incentive.

Best wishes to you.

Sincerely,

Karen Davis, Ph.D.
Machipongo, Virginia

13

Dear New Vegan,

First, I want to honor your decision to become a vegan. Your choice may have been easy or difficult to make; you may feel supported by your family or friends, or they may be mystified by what you've done. If it's the last, you should know that these people love you, and what they think may have nothing to do with your decision *per se* and everything to do with the moral shock you've given them. Through making your choice, you're challenging everyone around you to recognize that we are conscious beings with options in our lives: whether to live healthfully or not; whether to endorse unkindness and suffering or commit to nonviolence and compassion; whether to pay attention or be heedless. It may not feel like it at the moment, but the recognition that we have a choice in these matters is an enormous gift you've presented to your loved ones.

Secondly, safeguard your heart. Don't judge yourself by your own or others' expectations. Becoming a vegan won't solve your problems. It won't necessarily make you better-looking, more successful, or smarter. Voices will urge you to do more, be purer, work harder for the cause. They may criticize you for your inadequacies and make you feel guilty at not changing the world immediately. One of those voices may be your own. With all that you know, and all you'll continue to learn, it's easy to burn out, become overwhelmed, fall silent. That's why you need to protect yourself.

You are one among legions of people over the centuries who've tried to live lightly on this planet and care for the discarded and mistreated. Some folks were famous, others unknown; some of their achievements are recorded, others are lost to history. Whether you've heard of your forebears or not, it doesn't matter: they all made a difference in their own way. They had moments of doubt, even despair, at the slowness of change and the viciousness of our species. But they nonetheless trod the path you now follow, as others will after you. It's nobody's business but your own how you bring your talents to this movement. Take pride in your efforts on behalf of others: motivate, don't scold; challenge, don't shame. As Gandhi advocated, be the change you wish to see in the world.

Thirdly, follow your bliss. Enjoy food, cherish your body, make money, get a job, fall in love, have children—whatever your soul and your conscience demand. Veganism is about taking on life as well as renunciation, pleasure as well as discipline, the expressing of joy as well as the acknowledgment of suffering. Embrace your authentic self, because by being truly yourself you'll lead a whole life championing nonviolence rather than butting your head against the constraints of an imagined notion of what being a vegan means. After all, fighting for compassion and against cruelty should start with yourself: if you've no love for who you've become, why would anyone want to join you on the vegan journey?

Finally, *always* remember who you were before you chose veganism, and what combination of factors encouraged you to change. In doing so, you'll carry with you the necessary humility, thoughtfulness, and capacity to listen that will enable you to awaken others to veganism, just as you were awakened.

Martin Rowe
Brooklyn, New York

14

Dear New Vegan,

I would first like to say thank you, and welcome. Thank you for choosing compassion. It should be the norm, but it is not, so your choice is extraordinary. You may find that sometimes this choice won't be easy to adhere to, but your conscience will be at peace if you stick to your convictions.

It is important to surround yourself with support. I found it helpful to subscribe to vegan magazines, and read all the books I could. If I ever needed inspiration, I would re-read my books, skim vegan blogs, and watch YouTube videos. I also found it helpful to join a potluck group where I could be surrounded by other supportive vegans and discuss topics that would be difficult to discuss with non-vegans. It is also wonderful to attend gatherings where all the food is vegan.

The vegan message is spreading, and our community is growing every day. I hope you find this peaceful way of living as life-enhancing as I have. Thank you for opening your mind and your heart and choosing to be vegan.

Jennifer Gloodt
Joliet, Illinois

15

Dear New Vegan,

Your journey led you to these pages of support, hope, insight, compassion, love, understanding, and so much more. No matter how you ended up on this path, you are not alone. Please, never forget that.

My journey started back in 2002 as a freshman in high school. It started with a mouse. An innocent, sentient being I was told I had to dissect or I would fail. I was ridiculed by my peers. My teacher made fun of me in class. As I addressed the school board regarding my moral and ethical objections, my voice may have been shaky, but my purpose was clear. I was questioning, learning, growing. My mom stood by my side as I accepted my "F" and walked out of class on dissection day. We held a two-person demonstration and vigil on the sidewalk outside the school. I reached out to a local animal advocacy group and was soon standing beside compassionate people doing peaceful demonstrations. There on a sidewalk in St. Paul, my life changed forever. A woman named Anne asked me if I had ever personally known a cow or a pig or a goat or a chicken. I had not. She told me about an animal sanctuary she had interned with and worked for in California: Farm Sanctuary.

In the summer of 2007, I did a two-month internship at Farm Sanctuary, which I highly recommend to everyone. That internship (and the love of a goat named Chili) inspired me to move from Minnesota across the country to pursue a career as an animal caregiver. I spent four years of my early twenties caring for animals rescued from the animal agriculture industry. I cared for amazing animals alongside some truly amazing people. Caring for these animals is not an easy task. Some people believe that all I did all day is sit around and pet animals. My job was far from that. I took care of animals who were bred and manipulated to increase the mass of their muscles or their egg laying or milk production to make people more money. These animals were bred for extremely fast growth and very short lives. I have seen hens come to us with their beaks cut off, their bodies featherless. I have watched male calves—seen by the dairy industry as trash—try to nurse on anything they could find, because they had no mom to nurse from. I held a turkey—whose legs could no longer support her weight—as she was euthanized. She was barely a year old.

I have seen a lot of sad things, heartbreaking things, things that make me ashamed to be a human being. . . . I have also had the joy of witnessing individual animals—once part of a faceless crowd—literally come to life. I watched as they experienced many firsts in their lives: lying in the sun, stretching their wings, building a nest. I know each of them by name. They fill me with memories of healing, forgiveness, and joy. I will carry them with me for the rest of my days.

New Vegan, I need to share with you a story of a chicken who forever left a mark on my soul. I cannot tell you the moment our friendship began or how it really started. I just looked and there she was, one of the sweetest faces I have ever seen, standing near my side with the leg band number 28. I looked her up in our sanctuary log and learned her name was Andy. She came to Farm Sanctuary after being rescued from an "organic free range" farm. The girls rescued from that place had embedded leg bands.

Andy didn't have the deep scar on her legs as many of the others did. She was a chicken who kept mainly to herself and seemed off in her own little world at times. Whenever I was in the chicken barn I would call out her name, and if she wasn't busy she came running up to me. I would pick her up and hold her close to my chest, gently petting her. On days when I had more time or on my breaks I would sit down and let her jump on my lap. Sometimes, she just wanted some company; other times she would snuggle in for a little nap. I rubbed her cheeks and chin as her eyes slowly drifted shut. I encouraged other people to start calling out to Andy, but she didn't come to everybody. She clearly had her favorite people. I feel very honored and grateful she allowed me to be her friend.

For every animal I have known and cared for, I have a story. Every animal is an individual. They all express fear and avoid pain. Each has feelings and preferences. They all enjoy food and sunshine, the earth, and friends. Behind each animal I have known are billions of animals who will never be known to anyone . . . even themselves.

New Vegan, you are not alone. You stand for these animals. You stand for Andy. You stand for compassion and wisdom and justice. You stand among the very best of human beings.

With Compassion,

Ashley Curtis
Davis, California

16

Dear New Vegan,

Be sure to have people in your life who care about what you care about.

You see, I've been vegan twice. There's a lot of rancor in the animal rights community about "ex-vegans," but I know how easy it is to forget who you are.

I went vegan as a young adult for all the right reasons. I was an activist, and became friends with other activists who worked for nonhuman animals. I listened to them, did reading and research and thinking of my own, and quickly went vegetarian and then vegan. Going vegan was a challenge, but a good one. I had to learn to cook, which is a practice I grew to love. I worked on campaigns that connected animal rights, feminism, and peace activism, and was thrilled by learning about the ties between these efforts. The group of animal rights activists I worked with were queer, victims of sexual and domestic abuse, recovering drug addicts, and poor. The long meetings that were required for us to agree and make decisions together drove me bananas, but I *learned*, and these were solidly and fiercely "my people."

When I moved across the country to attend graduate school, I landed in a different world. The pace on the east coast was faster, more relentless. My colleagues' understanding of how to succeed, or even how to survive, was different from mine. I was the only person I knew in all of New Jersey who got around on foot. I didn't know one single other vegetarian. People discussed racism and classism and feminism, but never animals. I was unhappy in my new environment, and eventually depressed. I was also broke. A year or so in, I started buying $.99 slices of cheese pizza and peeling the cheese off before I ate them. Eventually, I left the cheese.

I had been vegan and an animal rights activist for several years, and loved it, and then I just wasn't anymore. I was still an activist, spending some of the most fiercely concentrated years of my life involved with AIDS and queer activism in NYC.

All the things I had believed and felt as an animal rights activist were still with me. I hadn't forgotten, for example, the toll that milk and eggs took on the bodies of cows and chickens, the forced pregnancies, the drugs, the stealing of children, the injuries, and the premature deaths. But I also wasn't thinking about nonhuman animals as foreground subjects. They were somewhere in my head, but conveniently fogged.

One of the reasons I ended up with my girlfriend is because we both love animals. She was a part of my AIDS and queer work in NYC, part of the group I worked so tirelessly with. She, unlike the others, had done animal rights activism in the past. She, like me, lived with cats she adored. She knew what vegan meant. After a few years together, we, with several of our friends, attended an activist training camp. She and I had been thinking about going vegan, leaning toward it, dabbling. The camp was all vegetarian and mostly vegan, and we decided to spend the three weeks eating all vegan.

The cooks at the camp were fabulous, and everyone was amazed by the three big, wonderful meals a day they were able to produce on hot plates under a tent erected in a swamp. We were impressed by how little waste they created. Everyone, that is, except for two men attending the camp from New York who felt that the vegetarian menu was racist. These were the same two men we'd had a talk with at the pool because they'd thought we wouldn't understand their homophobic slurs in Spanish. They started bringing in meat dishes at each meal, in Styrofoam containers, to share with others who might feel culturally challenged by the vegetarian camp. The camp's scheduled activities ground to a halt for the last four days, and all we did was discuss this: vegetarianism and racism.

My girlfriend is from Brazil, and there were several other Brazilians at the camp from Mato Grosso, the area of the country most devastated by the beef industry. There were indigenous people at the camp who were vegetarian, and some who were *not*, but who viewed factory farming as unnatural and disrespectful, and would only eat wild caught animals after particular blessings and thanks. We talked about how slaughterhouse workers are often immigrants, and how dangerous those jobs are. We talked about environmental racism, about pig farming in rural North Carolina and cesspools of waste. We talked about how slavery and machismo were both cultural inheritances. We watched *Meet Your Meat*.

We "lost" that fight, in certain ways. Those activist training camps are no longer vegetarian, even though it cost them their kitchen staff and their impressive feminist-Iranian director. But my girlfriend and I committed to veganism then and there, unable to *not* be vegan with all the reasons in the forefront of our thoughts.

For the last dozen or so years, veganism has been second nature. This time, I've made sure to not only surround myself with other animal activists, but to regularly be around and know animals themselves. Volunteering at a farmed animal sanctuary has let me get to know and care for all kinds of animals that I'd not had access to: goats and cows and pigs and chickens and turkeys; to know their specific personalities, situations, and needs. Empathy flows much more easily when you communicate directly with animals. Caring for trap–neuter–release cat colonies reminds me every day what we are all up against: fighting to survive and be happy as best we can.

For me, this effort to be happy and survive includes remembering, every day, the things that we can do better, for animals, for the environment, for queer kids, for brown and black kids, for the differently abled, for sweatshop and slaughterhouse workers, for immigrants, for those living in poverty, for old people. In order to know who I am and be the best person I can, I can't forget that, for me, choosing vegan over and over every day means care for *all*. This means that I'm always learning, always needing to listen to others.

I sincerely hope this is what being vegan means to you, too, and that you will be fed by it.

Kara Davis
Beacon, New York

17

Dear New Vegan,

Thank you for choosing to listen when your heart told you that eating animals meant causing them to suffer greatly.

I remember being exactly where you are at this moment. And the "me" of today would tell the "me" of forty-odd years ago: "Don't let anyone tell you that it's wrong to feel exhilarated and determined— that's just someone's guilty conscience talking."

I first tried to stop eating meat when I was five years old. My family and I were staying in a little bungalow in a tiny town in France, and I loved playing with the chickens who roamed the grounds. One morning, I rounded a corner and saw a man cutting the head off one of my chicken friends. I was devastated. I ran crying to my mother and swore that I would never eat meat again, which I achieved for several days by not eating anything at all. My worried mother soon persuaded me to return to a "normal" diet. And for us, "normal" meant meat. Lots of meat.

My father was a meat-eater's meat-eater, and together we ate our way through the animal kingdom. We ate everything from wild boar and cockles to organ meats like liver and kidney. Like most adults and probably like you, I simply didn't make the connection between living animals, for whom I had nothing but love and respect, and the food that appeared on my plate.

But when I witnessed a group of snails destined for the dinner table cleverly escape from a paper grocery bag that they were trapped in, that same feeling that I had experienced as a five-year-old came rushing back. I stopped eating escargot. Then, on my next birthday, I ordered lobster. I had seen the animal alive and actually picked him out, but when he arrived on my plate dead, I suddenly realized that he had just been boiled alive for my fleeting gustatory pleasure, and I burst into tears. I never ate a lobster or a crab again.

Several years later, I was a law enforcement officer in Maryland and responding to calls about sick dogs and cats and wildlife—all the while eating triple-ground prime meat—when I came across a pig who had suffered horribly, and I had an "Aha!" moment. I realized that there was no difference between abusing a dog or a cat and abusing and killing a pig or a chicken. I knew then that it was time to stop eating meat. You, no doubt, experienced something similar.

My husband teased me about the decision and tried to tempt me by cooking wonderfully fragrant roast chicken. I sat him down and said, "You're supposed to love me. So that means you're supposed to support me. I'm not doing this because I don't like the taste of meat. I made this decision, which was hard for me, because I care about animals and I don't want to eat them anymore." I pressed on because, although I love the taste of meat, I love animals far, far more.

I didn't let my husband, my father, or anyone else discourage me, so please don't allow people to discourage you, either. You can explain to them, as I did, that if they care about you, it would help you if they would respect your feelings and your commitment to doing what you feel is right. And in my experience, people will not only come to accept your choice but also actually enjoy the vegan dishes that you make. They will see you flourishing and they will strive to be healthier themselves; they may even start to make changes in their own lives to be kinder to animals.

Not long after I went vegan, I started to feel that it wasn't enough just to empathize with animals. I had to put those feelings into action. I wanted things to change. I wanted people to stop using and abusing animals for their own ends, and I knew I had to do something about it. What I didn't know when I started People for the Ethical Treatment of Animals more than thirty years ago was that it would become the largest animal rights organization in the world. I had no idea that we would grow from five people in the spare room of my apartment to three million supporters. I had no way of knowing that we would win landmark victories for animals and that companies would change cruel practices because of PETA's campaigns.

When I first went vegan, I had no idea what it would lead to. You, too, may not know what fantastic things might happen because you stand up for what you believe in. But you know that you have made a change that you feel good about and that you want to make the world a better place. And you will. The world will be your oyster—when you stop eating them.

Sincerely,

Ingrid E. Newkirk
Norfolk, Virginia

18

Dear New Vegan,

This is the letter I never received. Who could have written it?

I was born in the midwestern U.S. into a middle-class, Eastern European, meat-and-potatoes family. The sound of breaded veal patties frying in a slick of vegetable oil on an electric stove defines the timbre of my childhood. Angular stacks of American cheese slices stuffed into a crisper with thin-cut salami, honey ham and pimento loaf, big-eye Swiss and Muenster and sharp cheddar by the block: indiscriminate textures, smells, and tastes. Never were there discussions about the food we ate—what it's made of, where it comes from. So long as the pantry burst forth with aging cans and boxes, so long as my plate was cleared at the end of each meal, then I could count myself fortunate.

For twenty-two years I consumed the bodies and byproducts of other animals, even three years after discovering an undercover video filmed on a mink farm in China; there I saw for the first time an atrocity of which I had been happily ignorant. The size, the imposing magnitude of that suffering (and the human violence underpinning it all), shocked me to new consciousness. I tell it to you now and the tears still well behind my eyes: a live mink, stripped of her fur while still conscious, and tossed into a pile of her brothers and sisters all writhing and looking up to the soot-gray sky, beyond the red and sinewy bellies and exposed veins of their brothers and sisters. This is what I will never be able to un-see.

The time it took for me to become fully vegan—a little more than three years and three hundred miles apart from that video—seems ever more mysterious and frustrating to me. A lifetime of self-intolerance and hatred alongside a formidable will to destroy myself filled those years to brimming. At the apex of it all I went away; I self-admitted to an eating-disorder treatment facility and exited, five weeks later, feeling manic and electrified and determined to reclaim the parts of my self that had been so grossly stunted in their becoming. I completed my undergraduate studies (replete with honors and a high-school English-teaching license, don't ask me how!), was pierced six times and tattooed twice in the span of a summer, and moved to Chicago to live with a hometown friend of mine who had been vegan for a year and immediately called into question my possession of cans of tuna and a half-gallon of skim milk. Again, circumstance opened me up to the curiosity and doubt that are invaluable to deeply knowing, and henceforth dismantling, institutionalized violence and the social structures and ideologies founded in and through them. I remembered the fur farm across the world and accepted that I could no longer allow myself to remain complicit.

Nick, my then-roommate (who is now my husband and proud fellow foster-parent to two Chicago street-cats, appropriately named Omar Khayyám and Burrito Hotcake, adopted almost immediately after I went vegan in January of 2010), handed me Jonathan Safran Foer's *Eating Animals* and advised that I read it carefully. (Know that this text is only a starting point: it has multiple pitfalls, questions left unasked, unanswered. But this is what we learn to do: to read critically, go forward in hopeful and serious critique, and to remain cognizant of the fact that although we cannot know everything we will have known nothing if we do not commit ourselves to read, and read widely and without pretense.) After finishing this book I accepted that I had no further excuse for suppressing the discomfort and the outright shame I felt for continuing to contribute to the exploitation and mass killing of other animals.

January 2015 marks the beginning of my fourth

year as a vegan. I have read unendingly and without remorse, actively engaged my mind and my body, and remained increasingly committed to this ethical and political stance. The extent of my personal, ethical, political, critical metamorphoses humbles and vitalizes me in my activism as an ethical-abolitionist vegan and radical eco-feminist. It is the will to say *no more, not in my name, never again in my name*.

But just what it *means* to assume such a rigorous and direct position of critique in this society I cannot fully tell. In spite of that, I have come to embrace and even to love my black-sheepness (which, as a female-bodied person, might have been my birthright all along): my embodied critique, the radical doubt evinced by my very presence at "normal" meals. Many non-vegans consider me an inconvenience to be "dealt with." This is true of self-proclaimed carnivores (omnivores) and, yes, even (and oftentimes especially) vegetarians.

In this new veganism of yours you'll likely be angry at first—for many of us, frighteningly so—but with steadfastness and growth comes a greater call to self-responsibility that will demand your humility and patience. That anger never truly fades, but sharp-edged hatred and intolerance *must* give way to heightened focus and determination. That exasperation you feel as a result of being undervalued, undercut, cut-through, and continuously silenced by those whose ideals and behaviors and traditions you call into question will disperse, with time. It becomes something else altogether: a warm calm, a settling you earn by coping successfully with life's abuses while remembering those times when you had no idea how (or if) you would make it through.

This is too much to write. I've asked myself over and over what to say to you and have ended up wishing that we could just sit and talk over tea or coffee because then we could digress and ask one another questions in real time. But, in the end, I want you to know that going vegan was perhaps the most important decision I have ever made in my twenty-six years of living. Thankfully, you are entering a community that is much larger, more diverse, and with more potential for affecting revolutionary change than ever before. It is a comforting thought.

In Solidarity,

Jacqueline Morr
Los Angeles, California

19

Dear New Vegan,

Welcome to Veganville! I arrived here New Year's Day 1994. There were maybe eight Whole Foods Markets in the world; no one would've believed they would in time become a key influencer on the grocery industry and a multi-billion-dollar company to boot. The Internet was text-based, with a good many online forums, and emailing—*if* you understood how to use it. So the world was rather different from what we see today.

Now options are soooooo plentiful—including the huge number of recipes available online for free with gorgeous pictures; the abundance of vegan cookbooks that continue to be published; dine-out menus noting what's vegan; and an ever-growing number of vegan food products becoming available in stores and online, too. The list goes well beyond stuffing our faces—well beyond. I am so happy for all these eating options making it that much easier to shift and live vegan! In the '90s, the concept of vegetarian was certainly familiar to many, although from my observation frequently disdained; and *vegan* was something most people simply didn't know about or thoroughly understand. That knowledge, however, steadily increased over these last two decades with PETA's work (whatever you think of PETA!) along with more and more printed materials showing animal abuse, factory-farm video footage, vegan forums and blogs, and eventually vegan documentaries.

It would be the '00s before I saw people regularly understanding what vegan was and connecting it to the idea of being a "strict vegetarian." And then I noticed something funny: people connecting this remotely familiar idea where monks and so forth lived as strict vegetarians following one of the ancient religious traditions—eating simple, clean, whole foods as part of their spiritual practice.

My life path has not led me to a monastery or any such thing. And yet, I too became vegan for spiritual and health reasons. This meant I shifted over to noticing what I was bringing into my body, and life all around. I reconsidered what it was to consume another mammal's milk meant to grow her young from some 70 to 200+ pounds in the first few weeks of life. I thought about what Nature is and what we might pretend it is. I began to consider how my food and life choices relate to the Earth's well-being: a healthier planet for all Life—animals, trees, humans, and all the rest. The shift in diet entailed reducing my consumption of negative energies, most especially murdered beings, for what might truly be a guilty pleasure. I no longer forced my body to labor harder during the most energy-heavy work it performs—digestion—by shifting to a cleaner, healthier, and benevolent way of eating.

Though I made this shift in my hometown of Chicago when it was still the meatpacking capital of the world, I had no resistance from family and friends about going vegan. Bewildered looks, for sure, though no resistance or misunderstanding. So it was open road for me. And I had one key supporter (repeated thanks, Kimberlie!) plus a generally divine ease about going vegan. And so it began.

It's good to remember veganism is and continues to be multicultural. Nearly every civilization has vegan foods at the center of their diet. From East Asia's ubiquitous rice, seitan (aka wheat meat), and tofu (aka [soy]bean curd) dishes to lentils from the Eastern Mediterranean and the Indian subcontinent, to quinoa, beans, and vegetables from South America and Africa.

Please believe and know that *veganism is for everyone.* It continues to frustrate and baffle me that some have not yet gained reasonable access to fresh vegetables, fruits, grains, and other whole foods.

Certainly that's a whole 'nother letter or book unto itself. Nevertheless, living a healthful, happy life seems more than a reasonable goal for all to have in this day and age considering the collective knowledge and wealth we possess—especially when easy access to eating plant-based food can be a potentially life-altering, planet-saving, animal-loving, violence-preventing, and soul-healing expression of love for All.

I do want to emphasize that you need to live *your* journey. It's not up to you to control another being's life, and of course that goes both ways. This is what the diversity of life is about, no? Embracing all that veganism has to offer, one honors the diversity of human and nonhuman life, and all of us continuing to live our lives. Best for your journey, New Vegan!

Demetrius Bagley
Astoria, New York

20

Dear New Vegan,

Welcome to the grand adventure! You've taken many positive steps in your life, but sometimes it takes years to see how important they were. With going vegan, you get to feel good on day one because you start saving animals with your first meal. If you have health concerns, you're likely to see a drop in blood pressure and cholesterol within a very short period of time. This is instant gratification in every good way.

You're making this shift at precisely the right time, whether you're seventeen or seventy. It can seem daunting. . . . What do I put where the meat/cheese/eggs used to be? Do I know all I need to about nutrition? How will I handle social situations? But it's really simple if you take it a day at a time. There's just a little you need to know to get started:

Eat Enough
The best answer to the ubiquitous "Where do you get your protein?" question is simply to eat enough whole, plant foods. The way to be deficient in protein—and in quite a bit else—is to either consume too few calories, or to eat almost all refined carbs or a fruit-exclusive diet.

Learn Something about Plant-based Nutrition

When you do, you'll know to eat a great deal of vegetables, fruits, legumes, whole grains, and some nuts and seeds, and whatever vegan processed foods you need to make this new way of eating easy, fun, and lasting. Eat some beans (or quinoa or pistachios) daily to be sure you're covered for the amino acid lysine. Consume lots of greens for a variety of reasons, one of which is calcium (non-dairy milks have as much or more calcium than cow's milk, too). If you're a young woman, pay attention to your iron levels; if they're low, eat foods rich in vitamin C along with iron-rich foods (greens, beans, grains) for better absorption; cook in cast iron; drink the water in which you've soaked dried fruit.

Supplement Wisely

Take vitamin B_{12}. Start now. It's not found in plant foods, and it's so hard to extract from any food that the Academy of Medicine (NIH) urges anyone over fifty to supplement B_{12}, regardless of what they're eating. Failure to do this could lead to irreversible nerve damage. Current thinking holds that a huge number of people, on every sort of diet, are low in vitamin D (we're supposed to get it from sun exposure, but we're also told to protect ourselves from the sun . . . can you spell "Catch 22"?). Get your levels checked and, if you're low, supplement with a vegan vitamin D_3. Many authorities also suggest that taking an algae-based EPA/DHA (readily absorbable omega-3) supplement for heart and brain health is also prudent.

Make This Absolutely Delightful

Add wonderful new foods and products and friends and experiences to your life every day. Discover produce you've never tried before at the farmers' market. Experience some novel cuisine at a Vietnamese or Ethiopian or Indian restaurant. Enjoy the respiratory relief of cleaning your house with natural, cruelty-free cleansers. Have fashionable fun replacing leather shoes and bags with vegan alternatives—not right this minute (unless you're very rich and feel like donating the leather and starting over); but when the time comes to buy something new, explore local and online outlets for vegan alternatives.

Do This for Every Reason

Anyone who comes to veganism has some particular motivation—to improve their health (or even save their life), lessen animal suffering, lighten the load on Mother Earth, or to stand in solidarity with those who lack enough to eat (due, in part at least, to the wastefulness of animal agriculture). Each one of these is the "right" reason to go vegan, but I encourage you to examine all of them. "Health" vegans are prone to returning to eating animal foods because "just this little bit won't hurt." That little bit, however, meant life or death to an animal. And animal-rights vegans sometimes neglect their own health. They see it as irrelevant, but fail to remember that each of us is an ambassador for this way of life, and people are observing to see how it's working for us.

"Love the People Who Wish You'd Just Eat Some Meat"

I used this as a chapter title in my book *Main Street Vegan*, because, after thirty years at this, I see that relating to others with love is perhaps the most important thing we can do. Accepting a person doesn't mean condoning what they do. Giving them room to be themselves allows them to, maybe, come to this way of life, or closer to it, in their own time. It's human nature to want to convert those closest to us, but sometimes we have the best luck influencing a coworker, an acquaintance, or a stranger on an airplane. Everybody else we can just keep loving—and always bring a really tasty dish to share.

Defy the Stereotypes

Whenever I welcome a new class of potential vegan lifestyle coaches and educators to Main Street Vegan Academy, I go around the circle and say, "Tell me what about you defies some vegan stereotype." I've heard, "I write country music," "I have a gun collection," "I've never lived with a companion animal," and "My favorite channel is FoxNews." Hurray! Veganism is about celebrating life—our own and that of animals and other people and the life of this living, breathing planet. It's not just for people who were at Woodstock, or who would have been if they'd been alive. We won't transform the lives of animals, get healthcare itself off the critical list, and make a revolutionary difference for all life on Earth if we're some narrow little group agreeing with one another on every detail. Every human being has physical arteries and a metaphorical, as well as a physical, heart. Self-preservation and empathy for others are universal human traits. When we realize that, we open the door to the vegan lifestyle to everybody who's curious about the adventure on which you've recently embarked.

Let's welcome them all. That's how, one of these days, we'll see the life-changing, life-saving wonder of a vegan world.

Victoria Moran
New York, New York

21

Dear New Vegan,

Congratulations on your decision! Welcome to the most empowering phase of your life.

The more you learn about veganism, the more you may feel frustrated that the world isn't as thoughtful as you are regarding choices for food, clothing, and other products. Please remember who you were last year. Were you not a kind, compassionate person, deserving of being loved? Give someone else that chance to learn.

Veganism isn't only about eating plants instead of animals. It's *ahimsa*, which is a Sanskrit word for nonharming. *Ahimsa* should also be expressed with positive action my dad taught as dynamic harmlessness, "Do the least harm and the most good." Think about your best qualities and skills. Think of something you can do today to benefit another person or animal. That is the *ahimsa* quality inherent in the vegan lifestyle—not just a diet!

Share the compassionate spirit and stay positive. The world is counting on our success, and the animals thank you.

For a compassionate world,

Anne Dinshah
Fredonia, New York

22

Dear New Vegan,

Welcome to the world of vegan living, in which your values of compassion and justice for all living beings are the foundation upon which you build your life. As a new vegan, you've taken a major step toward bringing your actions into alignment with your values. Through those actions, which are far more powerful than words, you have declared that what we do with our lives really matters—to ourselves, to other people, to animals, and to our beautiful planet. You have every right to feel very good about this.

Visionary author Will Tuttle describes veganism as "the natural flowering of consciousness freed from the continuous programming of the inherent violence in our culture. The word *vegan* is precious, inspiring, and demanding because it questions the core mentality of our culture, and it is the key to our culture's transformation and to its very survival."

When we become aware of the consequences of our actions and close the gap in our consciousness that blocked our empathy for the suffering of animals, veganism is the logical result. Compassion, harmlessness, respect for the worth and dignity of all living beings—and the commitment to bring our heart, mind, and body into every choice we make—these are the hallmarks of the vegan path.

Though there are powerful health and environmental reasons to go vegan, for us the heart of it all is that this decision, practiced like a silent prayer three times a day when we sit down to eat, is a moral choice about whether or not to cause unnecessary harm to innocent conscious beings whose lives matter as much to them as ours do to us. It's the Golden Rule personified: since we humans can lead happy and healthy lives without ever using products from animals, there is no moral justification to pay others to enslave and torture them while they live and then send them to be killed in a bloody slaughterhouse. When you stand up for the rights of animals, you are standing up for all that is good in humanity.

Our vegan journey began in June 2005 when, through a series of synchronistic events, we met Will Tuttle, who was about to publish his brilliant book, *The World Peace Diet*, and learned about the foundations of veganism directly from him. We also saw the eye-opening documentary film *Peaceable Kingdom*, and witnessed the immense suffering of animals raised for food. For the first time, we saw the agony of a mother cow and her calf when they are torn away from each other so that humans can drink the lactating mother's milk that, with all her heart, she wants to feed to her baby. If her baby calf is male, he will be sold and slaughtered for veal, while a female takes the place of her mother when the mother's milk production declines and she too is slaughtered.

The torture and pain that we witnessed routinely happening to farmed animals was so horrific that, as we drove home from the film, we agreed that we would never again contribute to such suffering. From that day on, we've been vegan, and we believe it is one of the best decisions of our lives. Sharing a commitment to compassionate living as a couple is a profound bond between us, and it has strengthened our relationship in a multitude of positive ways. Our only regret is that we didn't do it sooner.

Prior to becoming vegan, we cherished the companion animals who shared our home, but we'd never spent time with farmed animals, so we went to sanctuaries to meet them. It's been truly life-changing to hug a sheep, rub a pig's belly, scratch a cow's face, kiss a llama, hold a rooster, caress a goat, feel the incredible softness of a chicken's feathers, and celebrate Thanksgiving with living turkeys.

We now understand that these animals are as fully developed individuals as the cats and dogs we love, that they are "someone, not something," and that their lives are just as precious. As Joanna Lucas of Peaceful Prairie Sanctuary so eloquently states, "The value of a sentient life is not measured in its utility to others, but in its immense, irreplaceable value to the being whose life it is."

When you visit a sanctuary and meet the animal ambassadors, look deeply into their eyes until you see the unique individual before you. Admire their beauty; observe their social interactions; learn their stories; appreciate their joy in having fresh air, nutritious food, and the freedom to experience their natural behaviors. Despite enduring abject suffering at the hands of humans, these animals are able to forgive, trust, and befriend humans, once they've experienced the loving care of a sanctuary.

As you connect with these vibrant beings, remember that each one of them represents millions of others much like themselves, who also have personalities, individual life stories, friends, families, and an innate desire to live, but whose lives were filled with misery before they were or will be brutally cut short in a slaughterhouse. Make your remembrance of the sanctuary animals you meet a touchstone for grounding you in your commitment to refrain from any action that would cause harm to any of these precious beings.

Our experiences at Peaceful Prairie Sanctuary, Poplar Spring Sanctuary, United Poultry Concerns, Farm Sanctuary, and others inspired us to find artistic ways to be a voice for animals. Upon returning from a visit to Peaceful Prairie, Daniel wrote "Sanctuary Song," his first new song in several years. He then wrote "Justice," to share the true story of a magnificent rescued cow we met there, followed soon thereafter by several other songs for animals, which can be heard on his album *Songs for Animals, People and the Earth* (danielredwoodsongs.com). Beth uses photography as a tool to share the heart-opening beauty and personalities of the individuals we meet, with the hope that looking into their faces will inspire others to go vegan. (Her photos can be viewed at bethlilyredwood.com.)

As you begin your vegan journey, you'll soon find that you are not alone; many others have gone before you and provided everything you need for an accessible, informed, delicious, nutritious, and vibrant vegan life. There's a supportive vegan community to be found through Meetups, social media, online, and at conferences all over the country. There are countless excellent books, cookbooks, and videos to help you along the way. A few of our favorite resources are the teachings of Drs. Will Tuttle, Melanie Joy, Karen Davis, Neal Barnard, Michael Greger, Jonathan Balcombe, and Richard Oppenlander, as well as Norm Phelps, Colleen Patrick-Goudreau, and Our Hen House.

There's a powerful, inspiring vision we hold in our hearts of a benevolent, vegan world infused with love—where peace, compassion, generosity, and sustainable abundance nourish the lives of all beings. For this vision to become a reality requires a global transformation of consciousness. Every action based on love strengthens this transformation, moving it toward a moment of spiritual breakthrough. We believe this is especially true of actions on behalf of the animals whose lives depend on our staying true to our compassionate nature and, with our words and deeds, urging others to do the same. You, dear new vegan, can use your life as a force for good, bringing your caring, talents, wisdom, and sacred spirit to a cause that, in the fullness of its eventual maturity, will rise to heights that far exceed what any of us can yet envision.

With warmest best wishes,

Beth Lily Redwood and Daniel Redwood
Portland, Oregon

23

Dear New Vegan,

Congratulations on your decision to do what I consider the most powerful act a human can undertake for a kinder, cruelty-free existence and for the well-being of animals and Earth. You truly deserve praise and encouragement.

As a new vegan, you will face a great many ethical choices you may not have considered before.

What will you do with your old leather shoes?

Will you ride in a car with leather seats or sit on leather conference room chairs?

Will you demand that your romantic partner become vegan? Is vegetarianism adequate?

Will you attend catered functions or holiday meals where meat will be served?

What if you slip up and have a slice of non-vegan pizza?

Will you make sure every single item you purchase is cruelty-free and not tested on animals?

Will you have your tattoos removed, as most inks are animal-based?

Will you still squash a wasp trying to sting you?

Will you feed your cat meat or force her/him to

be a vegan, too, even though such a diet is potentially fatal to felines?

There are no easy answers to these questions. You don't even need to make all of your decisions at once. Ease into them. You may also find that, over time, your decisions may change. This happens to most, if not all, of us.

You have, however, now put the Vegan Target on. Your actions will be watched and scrutinized by many, including other vegans, some of whom will be negative and vocal. Regardless of your choice on issues like those I listed, someone will second-guess them. Someone will ridicule them. Someone will say you are wrong. Someone will say you are not doing enough. You will be called a hypocrite for not living an entirely cruelty-free life, which is, in fact, utterly impossible in our culture.

Make your own decisions about issues like these. Your choices will likely be different from those of other vegans around you; they should be or they wouldn't be your choices. Realize what this negativity is: a certain type of person—one who is not at peace with the violence s/he is committing in life—will feel a need to attack you and pick apart every decision you make in an effort to validate his/her own actions by undermining yours.

Remember that you chose this life to make the world a more peaceful place. Enjoy the sense of peace you will have from not adding your portion of violence and suffering to the world. Do not add suffering to your existence by listening to those who will undermine your efforts. When that person calls you a hypocrite for what s/he sees as a lapse, all you have to say is the truth: you're on your path, doing what you can, to the best of your ability. Even if you aren't meeting that person's idea of vegan perfection, you are still making every effort you can to create a more peaceful world. Do not add suffering by taking on that person's animosity, nor by attacking that person in return.

Imagine how beautiful things would be if we all did that.

Namaste,

Alexa McCormack
Milwaukee, Wisconsin

24

Dear New Vegan,

Relax. Is there whey in the crackers you just bought? Is there still a wool scarf in the hall closet, a pair of leather shoes under the bed? Relax! You won't have as joyful a transition if you're brittle.

You'll be surprised at what's challenging and what isn't. Your body and heart and mind will feel so damn good after a month or so that you'll probably be fine with "sacrificing" that beloved glazed doughnut. On the other hand, you may not have bargained for being cast in the role of Sample Vegan. You're representing veganism, the way each suffragist and civil rights worker had to stand in for their causes. And like them, the way you interact with the world makes a difference in how veganism is perceived. It's a weighty responsibility, and, like anybody, you just want to be YOU. Make sure you've got some people you can just be YOU around—it'll make the other experiences less tiresome.

Because we're role models, we create other vegans. That's a wonderful part of living a vegan life. But no one's going to want to join you if you seem miserable or angry, or if you make veganism look arduous or impossible. If someone sees you berate someone for eating that cracker, or asking a waiter seventeen questions and making snarky comments at the answers, or if you're unable to talk about anything but the horrors of factory farming, they will think that's what veganism is about and they'll run.

People will want to join you if you're a relaxed person who's joyful about the changes you've made and gentle with those who haven't made them yet. They'll want to join you if you have a sense of humor and enjoy your life. The pinch of whey in the cracker isn't what's making the world fall apart. Be patient and loving and quietly proud of the amazing person you are in the process of becoming. People will be drawn to that, and you'll help make more vegans. That will lead to a more beautiful world—and you'll have more people you can just be YOU around!

Gretchen Primack
Hurley, New York

25

Dear New Vegan,

Welcome to Planet Vega, where we eat nothing but iceberg lettuce and cardboard, and no one takes showers. (Ha ha.) But in all seriousness, here are just a few things I wish someone had told me when I first went vegan.

1. **The beginning may be hard.** Your family, close friends, and coworkers/peers will likely still be engaging with a deeply-rooted system of animal exploitation that no longer makes logical or ethical sense to you. This is hard—there is no getting around it. It helps to be prepared, because seeing someone you love and respect put a dead body in their mouth can suddenly be jarring. But please do not let your relationships suffer because of it. Remember that until recently, you, just like them, ate animal products, too. It did not make you, nor does it make them, bad people—not by any means. You will still learn from and grow with one another. The work that goes into truly understanding where the other person is coming from can only make your relationship stronger. And if you have the resources . . .

2. **Always share!** Sharing good food is my

favourite form of activism. When I went vegan in middle school, I wanted to tell everyone why. I mistakenly assumed that if only my loved ones knew what I was learning about factory farming, they would respond the same way I had and choose to stop supporting it. Well, turns out that if you talk about "rape racks" (the dairy industry's term) and pulverized baby chicks at the dinner table, it doesn't take long for no one to want to eat with you. On the other hand, if you show up at every social event with a hearty veggie stew, an irresistible batch of cookies, and a big smile on your face, you open up dialogue in a non-confrontational way. "Can I have your recipe? . . . Wait, you mean there's no dairy in this? Really? I didn't know something could still taste so good! Cool!"

3. **It will be even more fun than you expected.** I'm still blown away every day by the stunningly kind people I've met through the vegan / animal advocacy movement. Go to potlucks. Join discussion groups. Spend an afternoon leafleting with friends. You'll meet batches of wonderful, often quirky people to guide you. You'll laugh together; you'll cry together; you'll learn together; you'll make delicious desserts together; but most importantly, you'll support each other like none other.

4. **Remember to make time for self-care.** Please, please, please do your research on nutrition and make sure you are putting good things into your body that make you feel good. Remember that everyone's bodies are different, so something that works well for someone else might not be good for you, and vice versa. Do yoga, jog, meditate, play sports, go out with friends, journal, play music, find chocolate—whatever works for you to re-centre, refocus, and stay sane. And for the love of kale, please get your B_{12}.

5. **Please respect yourself.** I cannot emphasize this one enough. Sometimes just hearing that you don't consume animal products puts meat-eaters on the defensive, even if you have said nothing at all about how they should be living. When people's beliefs and/or habits are challenged, they sometimes say the strangest, even degrading things in an effort to convince themselves that you are too "extreme." (Personally, I have always found it puzzling that people regularly feed their children carcasses filled with cholesterol, carcinogens, hormones, pesticides, antibiotics, pus, and fecal matter, and then call others "extreme." But that's beside the point.) I have been assured that dogs do not feel pain, fish are not

animals, and my favourite, "You're gonna die!" (I actually think this person was genuinely concerned and confused. We had an interesting chat. I am pleased to report that many years later, I am thriving and very much alive.) Try not to let the absurdity get to you. An intelligent discussion to share different perspectives is great, but if it becomes clear that someone is just trying to provoke you into arguing, no response at all may be best. Remember that you do not have to engage. Just get together with a good friend and . . .

6. **Remember why you're vegan.** Sure, we've seen films of animal exploitation and read vegan outreach literature. We're familiar with the horror-film realities of factory farming, and we can quote the stunning statistics about torture, cholesterol, and methane until we're blue in the face. But when it comes down to it, we are social animals, and we need to connect with individuals. For me, there is nothing more powerful than visiting a sanctuary and mirroring a piglet's gleeful grin as she squirms into my arms for a belly rub. Make space for these moments. And most importantly, remember . . .

7. **You are not alone.** More and more people are embracing healthy veg living every day,

making connections and thriving with compassion, sustainability, and awareness. Welcome aboard the spaceship.

For the animals,

Madeleine Lifsey
Northampton, Massachusetts

26

Dear New Vegan,

Whether you like it or not, you now speak for all vegans, or at least that is what some people will assume. They'll ask you all kinds of ridiculous questions about desert islands, plants with feelings, protein, and how much you miss the taste of bacon. They'll tell you stories about how they could never give up cheese or about their friend who went vegan and got really sick or how eating meat is natural, whatever the hell that means. I know you probably didn't ask to be a vegan spokesperson, but now that you are, the way that you react to these questions could mean the difference between someone closing their heart and mind to the idea of veganism or leaving it open. With this in mind I would like to offer you a few pieces of advice.

Be accurate. First and foremost, please, please, please, try to steer clear of vegan dogma. When we make claims about veganism that are not (or have not yet been fully) supported by logic, science, peer-reviewed studies, etc., we allow others to let one bad apple spoil the barrel and dismiss the entirety of veganism because of one sloppy claim. Just because something is repeated does not mean that it is true, no matter how many people repeat it. Similarly, if something sounds good, feels good, or seems likely, that in itself is not enough to make it a fact. The good news is that many of the claims we make about veganism are ethical, and thus not necessarily dependent on facts. There is no need to know who came up with the concept of the Golden Rule to suggest it might apply to nonhumans. You can instead rely on logic, simple observations, and personal experiences (such as the idea that cats don't like it if you accidentally step on their tails) to make your point. Of course if you can also share some facts about a cat's brain and central nervous system, your argument may be even more effective, provided you can support your claims. So, check your facts, quote experts, cite sources, and when you give your opinion make sure it is labeled as such. These things are not difficult and they will go a long way toward non-vegans taking your position seriously.

Watch out for "recent convert syndrome." You've probably seen this with ex-smokers. A friend finally kicks the habit and they become the smoking police. They complain about second-hand smoke and rudely confront smokers about it. They aren't bad people; they are simply dealing with a gigantic change that they have made in their life (and good for them, by the way!) while the rest of the world continues on as if nothing happened. Your ex-smoker friend has finally found the strength to let the truth about their former habit win out over the addiction, and now that they have made the change they can't understand why everyone else doesn't do the same.

After your vegan epiphany, you probably felt the need to enlighten anyone who would listen, and probably experienced a fair amount of anger and frustration when people didn't seem very interested in listening. Try to remember that you were once one of those people who didn't listen. It may have taken you years to make your decision to become vegan, so you can't expect someone else to "get it" after a ten-minute lecture. I know you have passion for the cause, but often that enthusiasm can easily be interpreted as you being judgmental and accusatory. Instead, be nice. People like nice people. Would you join a group if the person trying to recruit you was pushy and angry? Well, maybe you would, but those groups are called mobs. Leave your pitchforks and torches at home and just be nice. It all comes back to the Golden Rule: before you went vegan, would you have preferred to be treated as an evil, ignorant, enemy of all sentient life, or would you have preferred civil discourse with someone who actually listened to your half of the conversation? Pretty simple when you think about it, right?

Be content with planting seeds. Simply by being vegan you are influencing the people around you. Every time somebody asks you about your veganism, you have an opportunity to move them in the direction of compassion or push them away. Try to be polite and respectful while they ask you all of their seemingly ridiculous questions about where you get your protein or how you could ever give up cheese. They may actually be curious about these things, and if they aren't, I have found that answering these questions honestly (and without sarcasm) can turn a question asked in jest into a meaningful conversation. They may not go vegan the next day, but in time the seed you planted may grow.

Don't forget humans. One last thing: now that you are vegan, please don't stop there. One popular criticism of vegans is that they only care about (nonhuman) animals. There are many ways in which we humans exploit each other. In the same way that vegans see little distinction between slaughtering an animal for food or paying someone to do it for you, there are many "hidden" instances of abuse in which we participate every day. That $10 pair of all-synthetic material shoes may sound like a great deal, but if they were made by underpaid or under-aged workers in a dangerous factory, perhaps they are not as vegan as they appear. It never hurts to look deeper and re-examine your own choices, and I encourage you to do so as much as possible.

Daniel A. Earle
Ann Arbor, Michigan

27

Dear New Vegan,

It is an honor to welcome you as you embark on what is most assuredly going to be one of the most transformative and significant journeys of your life.

I am thirty-four years old. I've been a vegetarian since I was twelve years old and vegan for the last six years. When I first transitioned to being vegan, I remember focusing a lot on the idea of *what I can't eat*. Meat was already out, and gelatin. Now came dairy and eggs. Whey. Casein. How about honey? Animal-derived products lurked everywhere, rendering so many seemingly vegan things off-limits. It was overwhelming.

When I finally got the hang of *what I can't* eat, I turned to the question of *what I can't wear*. Leather, out, and obviously fur. How about wool? Angora? Silk? Do I stop wearing things I already own? As for new things—what if it's recycled? A hand-me-down? A gift? And is it really better to buy crappy made-in-China synthetic shoes that wear out in six months instead of a sturdy pair of leather boots that may last a decade?

When I thought I'd gotten the hang of *what I can't eat or wear*, I focused on *what I can't do*. This was (and still is) hard. Horseback riding? Visiting zoos? Watching a dolphin show? Keep feeding my cats meat-based kibble?

What I want to share with you is that being vegan is a task worth pursuing, though you will never achieve perfection, not fully. Not because the temptation to eat cheese is so great, but because the world most of us live in is so bound up with the exploitation of animals that unraveling our own relationship to that exploitation is a truly monumental task.

To me, being vegan is about being joyful, gentle, and compassionate in my interactions with the world. That includes nonhuman animals, of course, but also plants, rivers, oceans, mountains, moss, lichen, and stone. And it includes myself.

Eating a plant-based diet, I'm happy to say, is the easy part. I no longer think of my diet in terms of *what I can't eat*, but in terms of *what I want to eat*. And what I want to eat is food that is *joyful*. Because eating, to me, is one of the most wondrous and joyful activities of being alive. And the Earth is brimming with the most magical flowers, stems, stalks, roots, seeds, nuts, and leaves. And to taste them is to taste joy. Seeking out plates filled with *joy* and that are devoid of *suffering* is, I think, the true goal of any vegan. Because yes, in the abstract cheese may taste good, and so may bacon and everything else your friends will be astounded you are "missing," but food is not something we can eat *in the abstract*. Because even if it comes to you from a grocery store aisle wrapped in plastic and glimmering in its sterility, that cheese or bacon really did come from a living, breathing animal who suffered mightily to end up in that shrink-wrapped state.

For me, pursuing the goal of eating joyfully has led me to seek out not only exclusively plant-based food, but food that has been grown, harvested, and manufactured in ways that minimize suffering. Eating joyfully takes a great deal of focus and intentionality.

I will be the first to tell you that eating joyfully is necessarily an aspirational goal, for it is impossible to avoid all suffering from sneaking onto our plates. The way I see it, there is no such thing as purely vegan food; there are animals lurking in every bite of spinach we will ever take. There are the bees and other insects who fertilized the crops. The farm animals whose manure became compost for my organic veggies. Crops are grown on farmlands that likely used to be forests and glens, killing off countless indigenous plants and rendering unknowable numbers of wild animals homeless.

Yes, there is suffering everywhere, and to be alive and human and living in an industrialized country means that we will take part in perpetuating that suffering. But to me this is not a reason to give up—because "it's too hard."

There is a Buddhist saying—a *meal gatha*, to be specific—that says, "Seventy-two labors brought us this food; we should know how it comes to us." I try to think about that *gatha* before I eat, and to thank the sun, rain, wind, soil, seeds, insects, birds, farmers, pilots, deliverymen, grocery store stockers, cashiers, and so many more—everyone and everything that labored to bring me my food. And with each bite, I endeavor to eat with intention, gratitude, and joy.

Beyond embracing a plant-based diet is a dizzying cascade of truly hard decisions, the ones for which there is no right answer. Each of us must reflect on and be open to the idea that our ideas may change and evolve over time. *Would I ever date a non-vegan? Will I allow a guest to bring non-vegan products into my home? Will my dog be vegan? My cat? My child? Even on Halloween?*

Being vegan, for me, has opened up a world of joy, love, and compassion for all living things. It has opened up a world of contradictions and frustrations, of difficult conversations and even more difficult choices. It has introduced me to a vibrant and diverse community, and has led me to feel ostracized from others I sometimes miss being a part of. It has made life both easier and harder, and it has made me think about everything and everyone differently.

More than anything, being vegan has been and continues to be a most extraordinary journey, one that I travel on roads real and imagined, through both the physical world and the winding streets of my most inner self. I welcome you to this journey, and wish you joy and gentleness as you navigate through it.

Iselin Gambert
Washington, D.C.

28

Dear New Vegan,

I've put off writing you this letter for a long time. Months, actually. Because I want to give you encouraging, inspirational words. But something in me just can't. I feel like what I really want to tell you is the other stuff. The ugly stuff. No sugar coating.

Be honest. That's what they told us to do when this project was explained. Be honest. . . . Well. . . .

Honestly? Being a vegan sucks sometimes. Sometimes, it's really, really f*ing hard.

Now, I don't know why you've chosen to be a vegan. Maybe for health reasons. Or political reasons. Or environmental reasons. Or maybe someone triple-dog-dared you. Or someone bet you couldn't do it, and now you have a lot of money riding on it. . . . But if you became a vegan for the same reasons I did, then the challenges you face will be many. If you became a vegan because you love animals, your journey will be hard.

It doesn't suck for the reasons you may anticipate. I don't miss cheese, which is mind-blowing. My ideal date night two years ago was trolling the cheese counter at Whole Foods. My boyfriend and I would drive one hundred miles, over a mountain pass, to go shopping for cheese at Whole Foods on date night! In fact, I actually decided to date him because he cooked me a super cheesy lasagna one night. And I kid you not—I cried. It was so f*ing delicious. And I can honestly tell you—I don't miss cheese. I don't know why. It defies science. I just don't. What I miss is being able to enjoy my dinner and not feel emotionally disturbed by what everyone else is eating. . . .

When you change your lifestyle to support your new, moral foundation that eating animals is not okay, you challenge what other people believe. When you sit down at Thanksgiving, and your grandma is upset that you won't eat her turkey—that sucks. When the centerpiece on the table is a symbol of joy and tradition to your family, and it reminds you of mass slaughter and suffering—that sucks. When you log onto Barnivore.com and find out the wine on the table isn't vegan—that really sucks. When your dad gets hammered and offers your boyfriend $100,000 to "turn you normal again"—that's kind of amusing. But it also sucks.

There will be no lack of bacon jokes as people discover and react to the choice you've made. And it gets old really, really fast. And then it makes you angry. And that also sucks.

When you go to the grocery store and walk past the giant, refrigerated meat aisle, and you realize all those wings, and legs, and chops, and rounds, and bacon, and deli slices are individuals who suffered greatly before they became food—that sucks.

When your roommate invites her mom to visit, and she makes you a vegan meal for dinner, and it has fish and butter and cream in it because she thinks it's okay if it's "mostly vegan"—yeah. . . .

Being aware of how many animals are unnecessarily suffering, and how normal it is, and how many people you love and care about contribute directly to that suffering—sucks. So f*ing hard. Because you can't force others to believe what you do. In our world, where it is normal to be raised on food carved out of the bodies of living, feeling things, it is often considered "extreme" to believe another lifestyle is healthy, or enjoyable, or "better."

Honestly? I told people I was going vegan by posting it as a Facebook status. I didn't want to try to explain it to my family. I occasionally will post things about being vegan on my page, but I almost never post Mercy for Animals videos, or undercover investigations, or the things that made me want to become vegan, because if I tell my friends and family everything I know now, and they don't make the same choices that I did—if they choose to remain ignorant or decide not to care—I won't be able to handle it. I'll be so f*ing mad. I'm fairly certain it will ruin some very important relationships. Because I care about it so much. Maybe I care about it too much. But only because so many others don't care at all. . . . It's really hard to let yourself care. Most people don't *want* to care. They don't *want* to change. Change is hard. And caring can hurt.

But! It can deepen your experiences and give purpose to your life in ways you couldn't anticipate.

There are entire ethnicities of food you've probably never had before that will blow your face off with deliciousness. There are moments you'll share with animals that will haunt you because of their beauty. You will discover new passions and make new friends. You will know one day, when being vegan isn't seen as weird or extreme anymore, that you were there when the world was changing. You were a part of a movement. Your choices mattered. You saved lives. You helped make the world a better place. And when you find your voice, and are moved to share your story with others and inspire them to change, you will get to feel the sweet satisfaction that you helped to build an army of compassionate soldiers.

My advice?

Learn. Always keep learning. Read more books. Follow more blogs. Try new recipes. Watch documentaries. Visit a sanctuary. Check out new restaurants. Ask more questions. And share what you discover with others. The only reason why being a vegan can suck so much is because the rest of the world hasn't caught on yet. Spread the love. With no shame. And watch it catch like wildfire!

When you choose to be vegan, you choose to be somebody's hero. A lot of somebodies, actually. There is nothing that sucks about that. . . .

All my love to you, New Friend.

Maddie Cartwright
New York, New York

29

Dear New Vegan,

Congratulations! In becoming vegan, you are joining a rapidly growing community of kind-hearted, patient, and above all supportive people. While people may not become vegan to find community, they could not find a better community by becoming vegan.

Until vegans are no longer a minority, however, a vegan may feel different, and she or he will need to decide how and when, or if, to speak up for animals.

To me, one challenge of being vegan is the challenge of feeling different. When I was younger, this did not bother me. I was happy to be "an environmentalist," gaining awareness of animal rights issues by canvassing for Greenpeace just out of college. I also learned a lot from PETA at that time, an organization whose radicalism attracted me. I was righteous and bold then, having once told someone wearing a fur coat on a bus in Chicago that I didn't approve of her choice.

Then, fueled by classes in Marxist and feminist ideology, I committed to "critiquing bourgeois hegemony" in graduate school—whatever that meant. I marched forward, often blindly, thinking about my life in terms of these commitments, rather than in terms of career or, more importantly, in terms of building human relationships.

These were mistakes. Even today, I think about lost opportunities for friendships that I could have formed through quiet conversations or by sympathetic inquiries about someone's life: simply by being a nice person.

Today, I am strongly committed to ending animal exploitation, and yet it bothers me to feel different, to be thought of as difficult or judgmental, because I truly am not. Thus for me, in my everyday life (when I am not doing activist work), working with and making friends with people who are not (yet?) vegan is probably the most challenging thing about being vegan, because I want neither to be isolated nor to give in to fit in.

The difficulty then becomes deciding how to raise one's voice. After learning about some unspeakable abuse on a factory farm, I may mutter to myself for ten minutes. Often I will talk openly and angrily with trusted friends. But speaking to others can be a challenge. Such speaking out can alienate people, and you don't want to bother people to help you make amends.

But speaking out can also persuade. I always

remember that I committed to veganism because of my vocal, brave sister. And so I will sometimes tell someone "who doesn't want to hear about it" this story:

On a trip with my extended family to Disney World a few years ago, my sister brought along a copy of Gene Baur's *Farm Sanctuary*, which I read casually at first, then carefully as I waited in line for such attractions as The Pirates of the Caribbean or The Haunted Mansion. The effect was immediate (perhaps because I was simply being reminded of issues I already knew about): Reading the section on chicken production, I threw away the chicken strips I had just ordered. I have not eaten meat since. If my sister hadn't asked me to read this book, I might still be eating meat. Soon I was committed to veganism.

Still, I think it can be most productive to speak up when someone gives you the opportunity to do so. Potentially responsive people may say that they do not have the time, energy, or money to go vegan. I try to remember that at various points in my life, I would have agreed.

Immediately before my trip to Disney World, for example, I had slipped away from being mostly vegetarian. Isolated and poor, I was struggling mightily to finish my dissertation while working full-time, after I decided to stop teaching in my department. The Sylvan at which I was employed was next to an Arby's, so I would often shuffle in there after work—most frequently for curly fries, but occasionally for a roast beef sandwich as well. Convenience and hardship justified these poor choices, I told myself, as I pedaled home on a rickety bike, sad and tired.

But then I remember that as a poverty-stricken graduate student I had lived for a couple of years in vegetarian co-ops, eating no meat and drinking tons of soy milk. So it works to remind people that poor and tired and busy people can become vegan.

When people lament that they lack a sense of purpose, I might gently tell them that fighting to end animal exploitation gives my life purpose, suggesting that they, too, could find purpose in helping animals.

I remember that it is not easy being vegan, that remembering that animals are relentlessly tortured is quite a burden to shoulder. Of course, a vegan's suffering is nothing compared to what animals go through. But still, it can be difficult.

So I devised a coping strategy that incorporates my desire to get along with others. When I resent knowing and caring about issues when others don't,

I remember that I wasn't always vegan. Scanning through the sympathetic comments people make on Facebook threads related to animal welfare issues can help create a sense of community. Reading articles noting declines in fur sales or various timelines for banning gestation crates can help one remain optimistic. I manage sadness and frustration by talking to my sister, and to others, at the same time that I try to remember, for example, Ingrid Newkirk's impatience with sadness, and her penchant for action.

Mostly, when I am working or hanging out with people, not as an activist but certainly as a vegan who wants animal suffering to end now, I remember that, like everyone else, I am a flawed, ordinary person.

Perhaps these strategies will help you cope and be an effective activist. You will, of course, encounter your own set of challenges. And you are, of course, armed with your own stories and history to meet them. Thank you for helping to end animal suffering.

Sincerely,

Jean Forst
LaSalle, Illinois

30

Dear New Vegan,

My gentle reader, I hope this letter finds you well. This journey you are about to embark on is a deeply personal one, and we each find our own way. I have every confidence you will find yours.

Any change has its challenges at first. My husband and I refer to our "rookie mistakes" in our early vegan days, like forgetting to check if soy cheese had casein or failing to pack enough snacks on road trips. But being vegan is more than just what we choose to eat and not eat. In time, you'll come to realize that that is the easy part, and that there is pleasure and possibility in the foods we choose to sustain us. The difficult part lies within us—how do we find beauty, joy, and courage to counter the violence teeming around us? To be vegan is to choose to be awake in a world that has opted to snooze. It is not an end in itself, but a process, and at times, it can be lonely.

I grew up in an Indian vegetarian household in Rockland County in the suburbs of New York City. My childhood home smelled of cumin and coriander that soaked into my clothes and backpack and was transported into my locker at school.

"What's that smell?" a classmate asked one day as we grabbed our books between classes.

"I don't know." I said, embarrassed, as I shut my locker door and rushed off to class.

At home, we ate South Indian specialties. Soft, fluffy white *idlies* that I liked to drown in *sambar*. My fingers would mash basmati rice with just the liquid part of the peppery tamarind rasam, leaving the cilantro and tomatoes behind. But outside our home, my options were much more limited and far less stimulating.

In elementary school, I always brought a packed lunch. One day, I forgot my lunch and my teacher decided to buy me food in the cafeteria. They were serving hamburgers that day.

I motioned to my teacher to bend down so I could tell her something. I whispered to her that I didn't eat meat.

"What do you want on your bread then?" she yelped.

"Lettuce." Another whisper.

"What else besides lettuce?" she asked.

"Nothing," I said.

"You can't eat just that. That's rabbit food!" The little kids in line erupted with laughter.

Despite my desire to be "American" at this age,

I never wished to eat meat, but I didn't have the words to describe why not when bombarded with questions.

"Don't you want to know what it tastes like?" kids would ask me.

"No? Maybe that's because she's never tried it."

"You never ate meat in your life?"

"Not even by accident?"

All I could muster were yes/no responses, and for the most part I tried to keep my diet to myself. Back then, there were many things about myself I was discovering, many things I was uncertain about. As a first-generation American, I was reconciling my identity between two worlds, neither of which I felt I fully belonged to. But not eating animals was one thing I was sure of. In those early years, it seemed instinctual. In later years, it became informed. It was sometime in middle school when I made it clear, to myself more than anyone, that the decision was mine. I can't pinpoint a moment, just a shift in diction. A change in two letters.

"You can't eat meat?"

"I *won't* eat meat."

I moved out of the suburbs to New York City for college, which was liberating for many reasons, especially when it came to eating. I said goodbye to meals of iceberg-lettuce salads and fries, and began a series of adventures on my student budget based on two lovely words: "Lunch Special." In the years that followed, I read more books on animal agriculture. A former dairy farmer once told me how cows and their calves, once separated, would bellow, calling to each other throughout the night. I gave up ice cream.

At first, it was hard for my Hindu vegetarian parents to understand why I would avoid dairy, even though I was raised a strict vegetarian.

"Milk is OK. It doesn't harm the cow," they said. "We only take what is left over from the calf. We are helping the mother, by milking her."

"This isn't India," I told my parents. "That's not how it is here." (Years later, I began researching the Indian dairy industry and learned of its cruelties. But the treatment of cows was itself a sacred cow—too highly regarded to be questioned.)

I felt lucky to be awake. When I first went vegan, I wanted to know the truth about *everything*. It felt like a responsibility of planet citizenship. But knowing can be both empowering and paralyzing. It can feel like walking a tightrope between hope and despair.

If you find yourself at such an unsteady moment, know that you are not alone. You may feel overwhelmed carrying this burden, but I hope you come to realize what a wonderful gift it is to open yourself up to this compassion, and be sure to extend this kindness to yourself.

I try to find the part of me that had the courage to say, "I won't," many years ago. As a new vegan, you may not yet have the words to explain your choices, but there is something inside you that is guiding you. As Rilke said, go into yourself. Find that part of you—the best of you—and protect it. Someone once told me that hope is not something you have, but something you keep. I keep mine there.

Yours,

Sangamithra Iyer
Brooklyn, New York

31

Dear New Vegan,

The first thing I must say to you is that I am very, very proud of you. You have begun a journey that many people find very difficult to start and that most people never begin. I want to acknowledge your decision to begin while letting you know that you are experiencing the hardest leg of the trip.

To continue the analogy, you are in the phase of your trip where you're fumbling for your ticket, where people are looking at you incredulously while saying, "You're going where? Don't you know that veganism is _____?" where the blank is filled with "impossible," "unhealthy," "dangerous," "likely to hurt your mother's feelings," "a drop in the bucket," "a futile effort," "too weird," "against God's plan," and so on. You know why you're going, but you can't find the words to explain it fast enough or smoothly enough. And sometimes doubt creeps in, though you try to push it away.

That is where I come in. I want to be your traveling companion! I've been down this road and to this place, and it is now home, sweet home. I want you to feel the joy I've felt in coming to veganism. Of course, there is the despair that comes with opening one's eyes and really seeing the landscape for the very first time, but there is also catharsis in knowing that I no longer am complicit in the torture and death of my fellow beings who share the world with us. I want that for you!

I want you to meet all of my vegan friends. We will help you to find the ruts in the road so that you can avoid them; we'll point out the rainbow of color in the foods we eat; we'll hand you a vegan cupcake; and we'll be there for you to lean against when you're weary of the world as it is.

We're heading towards a better world, and you are now part of that peaceful push. We're so glad to have you with us as we come to a place where compassion, and justice, and love dwell. We'll get there. Our journey will end when all the world is vegan, and all beings will find refuge.

With hope, and love,

Linda Nelson
Pittsboro, North Carolina

32

Dear New Vegan,

Welcome to our amazing community.

Your new vegan life will be filled with great joy and infused with great heartbreak. As your journey continues, you'll discover more unimaginable and senseless cruelty than any one mind and heart can bear. You do not need to travel this path alone. Reach out and connect with other vegans. We can share our burdens and celebrate our milestones; we can find sanity in the insanity together.

Intentionally or unintentionally, three times a day, your plate is a protest against the cruel status quo. That's remarkable, except that not everyone at the table will appreciate your activism. Some may even interpret it as an inconvenient and senseless rebellion. It's strange: I know that peace starts on my plate, but who knew that my plate could start so many wars? Sadly, my choices often make people feel uncomfortable, defensive, or angry. And in turn, to avoid conflict, I wonder if I should remain silent when challenged or cushion the truth when questioned. But then I remember the animals. I remember that my voice—that our voices—are all they have. It's then that my convictions outweigh my fears of being labeled as the troublemaker, outcast, or fanatic. It's then that I realize I should never apologize for wanting to make the world a better place.

Being vegan means having compassion for all animals, including humans. Embrace others with the positivity, enthusiasm, and empathy that are the foundations of our cause. Most of us weren't born vegan, so tap into your pre-vegan self to understand how you got here and why you hadn't arrived sooner. Then, use that same kindness and patience with yourself as you continue to define and redefine your life. There is no such thing as the perfect vegan. There are only the kindest versions of ourselves we can gift to the world from moment to moment.

You are the change your world has been waiting for. Live proud. Love hard. Think bright.

Sincerely,

Angela Seiw
Toronto, Canada

Biographies

Demetrius Bagley is an award-winning producer of the documentary film *Vegucated* (2011) and the producer at Get Vegucated LLC.

Rick Bogle was a contented middle school teacher who, in 1997, became a full-time animal rights campaigner after parents threw a fit over his classroom rule forbidding the killing of the occasional insects who found their way into his classroom. He now lives in Madison, Wisconsin, with his wife, a cat, and a dog. He blogs at primateresearch.blogspot.com.

Maddie Cartwright is a playwright/actor/waitress currently residing in Brooklyn, New York. She loves coffee, the fall, and making her mom laugh. Her inspiration and partner in crime is an adopted bunny named Buttercup, who is always reminding Maddie why we should not eat, wear, test on, or toss out animals we no longer want. . . . We all deserve love. You can check out Maddie's blog about her vegan adventures at maddiebabble.wordpress.com.

Ashley Curtis spent four years as an Animal Caregiver at Farm Sanctuary in Orland, California. The animals and people she met there left a huge impact on her soul. Then, she worked for a year at Animal Place's Rescue Ranch program as an onsite Caregiver, watching rescued egg-laying hens learn how to be hens. Currently, Ashley is living in Northern California with her fiancé, John, their daughter Maya Magnolia, and their six rescued cat children. She is in college studying Nursing. She dreams of having her own flock of rescued hens.

Tracy Curtis has a degree in Nursing from the University of Minnesota and works at Children's Hospital in Minneapolis as a Pediatric Hematology/Oncology Nurse. She is the fortunate mother of four children who never let her get away with anything and challenge her to walk her talk. She is grateful for all the experiences in her life that have stretched and opened her and helped her grow . . . and forever grateful for the wise and beautiful souls in this world—animal and human—who nurtured the vegan seeds inside of her.

Kara Davis is managing director of Lantern Books. She is a street activist who got her start with the Sanctuary Movement as a teen in Arizona, and worked for many years with Act Up and Fed Up Queers in New York City. She is a proud volunteer at the Catskill Animal Sanctuary, and lives in a crumbling old house with her girlfriend and too many rescued cats. Kara is co-editor of *Defiant Daughters: 21 Women on Art, Activism, Animals, and The Sexual Politics of Meat* (Lantern Books, 2013).

Karen Davis, Ph.D. is the president and founder of United Poultry Concerns (http://www.upc-online.org), a nonprofit organization that promotes the compassionate and respectful treatment of domestic fowl and a vegan diet and lifestyle. She is the author of several books, including *Prisoned Chickens, Poisoned Eggs: An Inside Look at the Modern Poultry Industry* and *More Than a Meal: The Turkey in History, Myth, Ritual, and Reality*. Karen runs a sanctuary for rescued chickens at United Poultry Concerns in Machipongo, Virginia.

Jason Derry is a doctoral candidate in Communication Studies at the University of Denver, where he studies the ways people talk about the placement and positionality of the environment and animals to children. A researcher, educator, and advocate, he has worked with several groups in grassroots lobbying in Washington, has led nature hikes through the forests of Indiana, once sat in a tree dressed as an owl to talk about the importance of forests to second graders, and is now publishing a children's book to raise literacy and awareness for elephant orphans of the ivory trade. His favorite vegan food is olive tapenade and avocado on toast.

Born in 1969, **Anne Dinshah** is a lifelong vegan and daughter of American Vegan Society (AVS) founder H. Jay Dinshah and AVS current president Freya Dinshah. Jay and Anne coauthored the book *Powerful Vegan Messages*. Freya and Anne coauthored the cookbook *Apples, Bean Dip and Carrot Cake*.

Daniel Earle has been vegan since 2001, although he did not become active in outreach until 2007 when he got involved with the Students for Animal Rights activist group at Eastern Michigan University. Daniel currently works for the Animals and Society Institute doing administrative work and staff support. Daniel is a former employee of SASHA Farm Animal Sanctuary and continues to volunteer there on a weekly basis. He is also involved with other animal advocacy and vegan activist groups such as VegAnnArbor and VegMichigan.

Jean Forst earned a Ph.D. in English at the University of Illinois at Urbana-Champaign. She currently teaches (and loves teaching) at Sylvan and at Illinois Valley Community College. Her favorite thing in the world to do is to run dogs at her local shelter, Illinois Valley Animal Rescue.

Iselin Gambert is a longtime vegan living in Washington, D.C. Her great loves are cats, bicycles, cities, the Norwegian wilderness, marzipan, and all things chocolate.

Jennifer Gloodt is a vegan lifestyle coach, artist, and mother of four healthy vegan children. She lives with her husband and family in the suburbs of Chicago, and blogs as The Avocado Mama at www.avocadomama.com.

Lara Goodman is social worker and therapist in New York City. She speaks and writes in the Tibetan language and aspires to raise awareness of animal agriculture among Tibetans and other immigrant populations in the United States. She's in complete admiration of those who follow their heart for the good of others. Her home is vegan, down to the clothing her family wears.

Ruby Goodman is a nine-year-old passionate vegan. She was educated about the ethical dilemma of eating animal products, but was never forced to identify as vegan. She enjoyed certain non-vegan treats with her friends and family for years until one day she told her parents, "I just can't eat it without thinking of the brutality that led to it. I don't need it anymore. It actually grosses me out." Ruby aspires to grow into her role as a humane educator. She wants nothing more than to open a farm animal sanctuary one day. Her mom and dad may conspire to help this happen sooner than later.

Julie Hanan has been involved in animal rescue, animal welfare, and legislative lobbying for many years. She spent almost a decade as a big cat keeper for a nationally accredited wild cat sanctuary, gaining an intimate knowledge of the issues facing wild cats in particular. Being a vegan, she advocates a compassionate lifestyle for all animals, now with an emphasis on the reality of life for billions of factory-farmed animals. Her six rescued animals at home also provide constant inspiration for her published articles.

Sangamithra Iyer is a writer and engineer and the author of *The Lines We Draw* (Hen Press). She served as an editor of *Satya* magazine and is an Associate of the environmental action tank, Brighter Green. For more information about her writing visit www.sangamithraiyer.com.

Kara Kapelnikova is an animal rights activist who writes the blog VeganRabbit.com.

Shelley Kaplan is a longtime pediatric nurse practitioner and lactation consultant. She enjoys organic gardening, reading, and creating ceramic crafts. She lives with her vegan partner and four cats in Oregon.

Madeleine Lifsey is the co-founder and chair of Animal Advocates of Smith College. Former intern with Farm Sanctuary and The Humane League, she works in the Philosophy for Children movement, seeking to empower young children to explore challenging ethical questions. When not giving pigs belly rubs or discussing anthropocentrism with second-graders, Madeleine is often found in a yoga studio, hiking a mountain, or in the kitchen concocting anything involving raw chocolate.

Alexa McCormack is the Executive Director of Alliance for Animals and the Environment, Wisconsin's oldest statewide animal advocacy organization (www.allanimals.org).

Victoria Moran, HHC, AADP, is the author of *Main Street Vegan*, *The Love-Powered Diet*, and *The Good*

Karma Diet. She is the founder and director of Main Street Vegan Academy and the host of the Main Street Vegan show on Unity.FM. Find out more about her work at www.mainstreetvegan.net.

Jacqueline Morr is a writer, ethical-abolitionist vegan, activist, educator, and stargazer. She received her M.A. from New York University in May 2013 and intends to pursue a Ph.D. in Psychology. You can catch her reading critical theory or science fiction at the library most days. She is a recent transplant from Brooklyn all the way to Los Angeles, where she lives in the bottom half of a dusty duplex with her husband, their two feline companions, and her as-yet-unpublished manuscript.

Linda Nelson has mentored and provided cooking demonstrations for the Peace Advocacy Network's vegan pledge and serves on the board of the recently formed (but very busy) Triangle Chance for All Microsanctuary. She now has the chance to encourage others to live a vegan life while working with a team of very committed ethical vegans to rescue and provide lifelong sanctuary to a beautiful and growing flock of chickens. To work together with friends towards greater justice and love is what she has been seeking all along.

Ingrid E. Newkirk is the founder of People for the Ethical Treatment of Animals (PETA)—the largest animal rights organization in the world, with more than three million supporters—and is also the founder of all PETA's affiliates around the world. She is the author of 13 books, including *Making Kind Choices* and *The PETA Practical Guide to Animal Rights*. Her campaigns to promote cruelty-free living have made the front pages of virtually every newspaper in the U.S., India, and Europe.

Lynn Pauly is just one of the many vegan cheese heads living in Madison, Wisconsin. She has worked for several animal rights organizations such as In Defense of Animals, Primate Freedom Project, and Alliance for Animals. She lives with her husband, Rick Bogle, and their barking dog, Micky.

Gretchen Primack is the author of two poetry collections, *Kind* (Post-Traumatic Press, 2013), which is all about the dynamic between humans and other animals, and *Doris' Red Spaces* (Mayapple, 2014). She's also the co-author of *The Lucky Ones: My Passionate Fight for Farm Animals* (Penguin Avery, 2012) with Jenny Brown of Woodstock Farm Animal Sanctuary. Her poems have appeared in *The Paris Review*, *Prairie Schooner*, *The Massachusetts Review*, *FIELD*, *Antioch*

Review, Ploughshares, and other journals. Primack has worked as a union organizer, working women's advocate, and prison and jail educator. Her website is www.gretchenprimack.com.

Vegan since 2005, **Beth Lily Redwood** is a graphic designer, photographer, digital artist, and writer. She is the publications manager for Melanie Joy's Carnism Awareness and Action Network, a certified World Peace Diet Facilitator, and has a master's degree from the University of Wisconsin-Madison. Her art and photography can be viewed at bethlilyredwood.com. Beth's artwork, photography and/or writing have been featured in *The Missing Peace* by Judy Carman and Tina Volpe, *Turning Points in Compassion* by Gypsy Wulff, a National Museum of Animals and Society exhibit, on Our Hen House, in *Poultry Press* magazine, and in galleries.

Daniel Redwood is a singer-songwriter who has performed at the Animal Rights National Conference, Chicago VeganMania, the Conference for Animals and the Environment, and at Animal Place. His music was featured on Veganpalooza, and he has been interviewed on Main Street Vegan Radio and Radio Free Rescue. His reviews of animal rights books have been published on the Webby-winning Our Hen House website. Dr. Redwood practiced chiropractic for 25 years and is now Director of the Master of Science in Human Nutrition and Functional Medicine program at the University of Western States. He is an associate editor of *Topics in Integrative Healthcare*, a member of the editorial advisory board of the American Chiropractic Association, and was a founding board member of *The Journal of Alternative and Complementary Medicine*. An archive of his health writings can be found at redwoodhealthspeak.com.

Martin Rowe is the publisher at Lantern Books and the author of, among other books, *The Polar Bear in the Zoo: A Speculation* and *The Elephants in the Room: An Excavation*.

Kurt Schwemmer is a thirty-four-year-old, recently married, vegan. He enjoys hiking with his wonderful wife, Meri, his lifelong trail dog, Winnie, and his small dog with a big spirit, Lola. He's an electrical engineer, an outdoor adventurer, and an animal lover. Raised in the midwest eating meat, veganism was an unfamiliar choice. His love of his dog and recent popular media informing him of the health and environmental aspects of the diet led him to veganism.

Angela Seiw is an urban animal, outgoing introvert, and culinary activist. This curious and well-travelled earthling holds a Master of Education from the University of Toronto and a Vegetarian Cuisine Certificate from George Brown College. Angela works in corporate design and communications and owns Little Vegan Kitchen, a Toronto-based catering company focused on spreading vegan love through the stomach. She enjoys cat cuddles, quirky fonts, and vanilla bean speckles.

Keane Southard is a composer and pianist (keanesouthard.instantencore.com) who recently spent a year in Brazil as a Fulbright scholar doing research on music education. He has been vegan since 2010.

Mark Turner is a lifelong dog and cat lover. He retired early from a career in aviation medical sales to start a dog training business. At the same time, he began volunteering at a local dog and cat animal rescue shelter. A few years later, in January 2012, he finally made the connection between those animals who share our homes and those who do not. He now has his perfect job, as Head of Sales for a 100% vegan food company. He loves to travel, is an avid motorcyclist, and is on a quest to visit all fifty U.S. state capitol buildings by motorcycle. He lives in Chicago with his wife, to whom he has been married for more than twenty-five years.

About the Publisher

LANTERN BOOKS was founded in 1999 on the principle of living with a greater depth and commitment to the preservation of the natural world. In addition to publishing books on animal advocacy, vegetarianism, religion, and environmentalism, Lantern is dedicated to printing books in the United States on recycled paper and saving resources in day-to-day operations. Lantern is honored to be a recipient of the highest standard in environmentally responsible publishing from the Green Press Initiative.

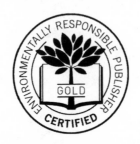

www.lanternbooks.com